THE WELLNESS
— COMPANY —

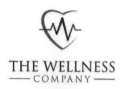

IN LOVING MEMORY OF
VLADIMIR ZELENKO, MD

| DR. RICHARD AMERLING, MD | DR. HEATHER GESSLING, MD | DR. PETER A. MCCULLOUGH, MD, MPH | DR HARVEY RISCH, MD, PHD | DR. JANA SCHMIDT, ND | DR. JEN VANDEWATER, PHARMD |

"Dr. Zelenko was a fierce fighter for truth and medical freedom. His legacy lives on through a core group of doctors who take their Hippocratic Oath to heart. In this book, six valiant doctors reveal their journey, their battles, and their compassion for the promotion of true health and wellness."

Lieutenant General Thomas G. McInerney, USAF (Ret.)

The Next Wave Is Brave

Standing Up for Medical Freedom

The Next Wave Is Brave

Standing Up for Medical Freedom

Foster Coulson
Richard Amerling, MD
Heather Gessling, MD
Peter McCullough, MD, MPH
Harvey Risch, MD, PhD
Jana Schmidt, ND
Jen VanDeWater, PharmD

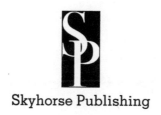

Skyhorse Publishing

Skyhorse Publishing books may be purchased in bulk at special discounts for sales promotion, corporate gifts, fund-raising, or educational purposes. Special editions can also be created to specifications. For details, contact the Special Sales Department, Skyhorse Publishing, 307 West 36th Street, 11th Floor, New York, NY 10018 or info@skyhorsepublishing.com.

Skyhorse® and Skyhorse Publishing® are registered trademarks of Skyhorse Publishing, Inc.®, a Delaware corporation.

Visit our website at www.skyhorsepublishing.com.

10 9 8 7 6 5 4 3 2 1

Library of Congress Control Number 2022917528

Hardcover ISBN: 978-1-5107-7668-5

Cover Design by Stephanie Pierucci
Edited by Stephanie Pierucci & Dale Chaplin

Printed in the United States of America

Contents

Publisher's Note xi

Other Important Notes.. xiii

Introduction: Bravery & the Future of Wellness...................... xvii

Dr. Heather Gessling 1

Chapter One: Finding Your Tribe... 3

Dr. Peter McCullough.. 31

Chapter Two: Preparing Your Heart for The Next Wave 33

Dr. Jen VanDeWater 67

Chapter Three: The Garden is Ripe 69

Dr. Harvey Risch 99

Chapter Four: Because of Science, We Can Be Brave....................... 101

Dr. Richard Amerling 129

Chapter 5: Conscious Medical Re-Education.................................. 131

Dr. Jana Schmidt.. 167

Chapter 6: Nature Holds the Key to Transforming Health.............. 169

Conclusion: A Call for Connection 191

Join The Wellness Revolution 201

Author's Note 205

Dedication

To Zev Zelenko (1973-2022)

This book is dedicated to a man who created the ripple that started the wave. Dr. Vladimir (Zev) Zelenko, your compassion, courage and serenity will never be forgotten. Thank you for illustrating that an "average country doctor" with a few stones in his slingshot can disarm a giant. We are honored to continue his fight until we decapitate the serpent…

Publisher's Note

PLEASE READ:

This book details the author's personal experiences and opinions about general health, prevention of disease, nutritional supplements, and/ or exercise. The author is not your healthcare provider. The Wellness Company Team including Dr. Richard Amerling, Dr. Heather Gessling, Dr. Peter McCullough, Dr. Harvey Risch, Dr. Jana Schmidt, and Dr. Jen VanDeWater as well as The Wellness Company are providing this book and its contents as a story on an "as is" basis with no representations or warranties of any kind with respect to this book or its contents. The authors and publisher disclaim all such representations and warranties including, for example, warranties of merchantability and healthcare for a particular purpose. In addition, the author and the publisher do not represent or warrant that the information accessible via this book is accurate, complete or current.

The statements made about products and services have not been evaluated by the U.S. Food and Drug Administration. They are not intended to diagnose, treat, cure, or prevent any condition or disease. Please consult with your own physician or healthcare specialist regarding the suggestions and recommendations made in this book. Except as specifically stated in this book, neither the authors, nor The Wellness

Company, nor any contributors or other representatives will be liable for damages arising out of or in connection with the use of this book. This is a comprehensive limitation of liability that applies to all damages of any kind, including (without limitation) compensatory; direct, indirect or consequential damages; loss of data, income or profit; loss of or damage to property and claims of third parties.

Understand that this book is not intended as a substitute for consultation with a licensed healthcare practitioner, such as your physician. Before you begin any healthcare program, or change your lifestyle in any way, you should consult your physician or another licensed healthcare practitioner to ensure that you are in good health and that the examples contained in this book will not harm you. This book provides content related to physical and/or health issues. As such, use of this book implies your acceptance of this disclaimer.

Other Important Notes

In this book we choose not to use the term vaccine when referring to the COVID-19 injection. This investigative vaccine does not work in the same way as conventional vaccines in that it does not prevent the illness, its intention is to reduce the symptoms. In addition, it has not undergone the rigorous testing of conventional and effective vaccines. For these and other reasons, we have chosen to change the term to Investigational Gene-Based Treatments in certain applicable instances or simply "vaccine."

"The Wellness Company was born out of necessity. By unequivocally and unapologetically standing up for medical freedom and the right to affordable and personalized health care, our company's vision champions the right to make one's own choices for their body."

Foster Coulson

THE WELLNESS COMPANY

HELPING PEOPLE AND HEALTHCARE PROFESSIONALS FREELY THRIVE

WELLNESS	PHARMACY	TELEMEDICINE	MARKETPLACE
RELIABLE & THOROUGH CONTENT PROVIDED BY OUR LICENSED HEALTHCARE PROVIDERS	THE FUTURE OF INDEPENDENT PHARMACY GIVING PATIENTS THE FLEXIBILITY OF SERVICE THEY DESERVE.	PASSIONATE DOCTORS AVAILABLE FOR APPOINTMENTS & CONSULTATIONS NO MATTER WHERE YOU ARE.	GROUND-BREAKING DIETARY PRODUCTS CREATED BY WORLD-RENOWN DOCTORS & SCIENTISTS.

FOUR WAYS WE'RE CONTRIBUTING TO MEDICAL FREEDOM.
WILL YOU JOIN US?

Introduction

Bravery & the Future of Wellness

"Over the last few years, it has become so obvious to me that evil is a very real threat. The change from believing that evil was an abstract concept to recognizing its very real influence in the world has shifted how I see everything."

JP Sears

The past few years have both infuriated and inspired me. Like so many of you, I entered an existential cave a few years ago, questioning everything I thought I knew about the world around me. The book you're reading is a result of those inquiries. As a brother, son, husband, and especially as a father, when I saw the world manifesting into a terrifying, oppressive place in 2020, I couldn't sit on my hands. I found satisfaction in knowing that although each question only begat more questions than answers, I was destined to be alive in this unique moment in time.

Amidst the myriad of questions, I still ask daily, I have learned this about myself:

I want to create a measurably more healthy, loving, and free world. Peddling widgets has no appeal to me, no matter how profitable I could make it.

1. I'm a warrior fighting for my kids and grandkids to live in a healthier, friendlier world than the one we've seen. I *will* upend the evil entities who profit by keeping you unwell.
2. Above all, I've learned that I can't do this alone. I need you. By the end of this book, you'll see exactly what I'll need you to do. Spoiler alert: it involves the happiest, healthiest version of you.

Thanks to the past few years of re-establishing my personal life goals and heart's calling, I now have a deafening sense of purpose. I now see that my calling to disrupt and reset the way we do wellness was instilled in me even as a child. I grew up with a mother who was deeply in tune with holistic health and her body's natural intelligence. She taught us how to care for our bodies holistically, rejecting the notion of immediately reaching for the medicine cabinet or an antibiotic at the first sign of illness.

Decades later, I watched my wife struggle with hormonal health issues stemming from a vaccine she was pressured to take at 17, one that has since had a formulation change. She is one of thousands or more vaccine-injured women in her age group who have suffered as a result of this same vaccine, many of whom have struggled with a vast array of health issues.

Steph and I are blessed with two gorgeous kids. Unfortunately, our son, now nine, received a routine childhood shot that compromised his health and rocked our world. She threw herself into finding alternatives to the standard medical care to help him from the time he was an excessively colicky baby; for nine years she has pioneered health sovereignty and personal responsibility in our home—two of the key lessons we'll learn about in this book. Happily, our daughter was born into a much more health-conscious environment and has, as a result, had fewer health struggles.

Today in our holistic home we always reach for herbs or tinctures before pharmaceutical medications, taking care of our bodies through exercise and nutrition, growing our own food, buying organic and non-

GMO foods when possible, and supporting our local farmers' market weekly to get the freshest possible food and support our local farmers. Steph even has a flock of Silkie chickens that eat an organic diet - including our kitchen scraps - and provide us with nutritious, organic eggs. We actively teach the importance of all of these things to our kids so that they too can develop self-sufficiency with their health. I suspect that they, too, will inherit the blessing my mother bestowed on my brother and me of health consciousness and sovereignty. But even more importantly, I hope my kids will grow up in a world that isn't so broken. And I'm putting my money where my mouth is.

The Problem Reveals the Plan

Over the years, I have watched the current broken medical system fail numerous relatives and dear friends. There has to be a better way.

Patients come before profits; my Chief Medical Board and I repeat this daily, sometimes hourly. Each human body isn't a bag of diseases that needs medication to survive. Our bodies are the results of our lifestyles, food choices, environment, relationships, and the care, or lack thereof, of our physicians or healers. Your health provider may only spend fifteen minutes talking to you annually; checking off boxes on a chart loaded with questions they're given from a hospital corporation or insurance company that has nothing to do with your symptoms or health goals. That's not putting the patient first. We'll talk about that in this book.

Alternatively, the care from your providers may be loving, holistic, and comprehensive; they may assess, diagnose, and treat your health based on hours of getting to know you and your family. Your provider may treat your body as a unique machine; one that is unlike any other on this Earth. He or she may cherish your individuality and base their recommendations on your individuality and personal goals. That's the system The Wellness Company wants for your unique body to live in; one where it's treated like it's one-of-a-kind. Because it is.

When I jump out of bed each morning, all I see in the day's sprint ahead of me is the opportunity to infuse more wellness into the world through entrepreneurship and the different facets of The Wellness Company, which you'll learn about through the doctors who've written this book. You've heard it said that entrepreneurship is one part ignorance and another part confidence? I'm an optimist, so I'll roll with the latter.

I'm confident that we can stop the industrial poisoning of people for profit.

I'm confident that we can stop the blanket prescribing of unnecessary medications that aren't appropriate for every unique vessel and human.

I'm confident that we will build Wellness Pharmacies and Virtual Medicine services that care for human thriving, not merely human surviving.

I'm confident that we will build a nationwide and eventually a worldwide team of physicians who are not shackled to a bottom line designed to bolster insurance company profits, but who are committed to deprescribing and restoring healthy homeostasis and immune systems to our Wellness Company family.

I'm confident that we can move away from the current system of hospitals that are not practicing patient-centered care, where doctors and nurses are treating patients as a number on a chart.

The medical industry is broken, it is corrupt in places, and it is time for radical change. That's why we're here. But the enemy has pervaded every aspect of our lives; our medicine cabinets, our wallets, our ability to live freely. So that's why we fight.

Now, you know more about me as an individual. You know what drives me and motivates me. Let's move on to why I have felt utterly compelled to will The Wellness Company into existence.

If I have learned anything over the last two years, it's that as much as I believe Good will ultimately triumph, we are all individually responsible to help shine the light and create good in the world.

To me, there are two types of people: those who sit and wait for something to change, and those who fight with everything they possess to create that change. Now is the time to band together and co-create the change we want and need to see.

This book, *The Next Wave Is Brave*, is written by a collection of people who I am truly honored and humbled to stand beside because they aren't talkers, they're doers. They are all fighting tooth and nail to create change in this world. They are not ones to stand on the sidelines and judge everybody else's plays; they're out on the field running for the goal every day - blood, sweat, and tears.

Sustainably Shaking Things Up…

Before I tell you about how we are going to co-create positive change in the Wellcare space, I am going to tell you a bit about my own journey over the past two years.

Even as a young kid I wanted to be Indiana Jones. I yearned to adventure and save the world– with a side of entrepreneurship and business. Thankfully my parents were supportive of my dreams, even when they seemed "too big" or wildly out of the box. They taught me that radical thinkers created everything we see around us; once even a chair was a wild idea. Everything you see comes from a thought, and from that thought somebody took action. My thoughts all revolve around creating a freer, more healthy world, and to manifest that thought, I will put everything on the line. I already did so once, which you'll read about in just a moment.

I've been an entrepreneur since I graduated high school, committed to work that creates a positive impact through the disruption of old systems. I have always gravitated towards impact companies that have the ability to create a better, more sustainable world for all of us. Some didn't quite work out, and others have soared with success.

However, I can proudly hold my head high knowing that, success or failure, I always put my heart and soul into anything I put my mind to. I don't regret the failures because the universe uses those lessons to make each subsequent endeavor better in its mysterious, mesmerizing way.

One mesmerizing event that changed the course of my life was the Amazonian wildfires in September of 2020. During that time I found myself negotiating fire suppression aid for Bolivia between the Canadian Prime Minister's office and the President of Bolivia's office. You cannot imagine the drama involved in heaving these two bureaucratic offices uphill. Regardless of all the red tape, we got the aid package signed and prepped for deployment to Bolivia.

I was to fly down in advance to meet the Minister and the Bolivian President and to ensure that operations would run smoothly from the first landing. Knowing the reputation of Bolivia as a whole, I cautiously brought some personal security with me.

Then, fate intervened. My originally scheduled security person fell sick and was unable to join me. I reached out to my contacts and was able to find a replacement; little did I know that he would become one of my best friends and business partners shortly down the line. Dave is the most stand-up, bad-ass, ex-Navy Seal you can imagine; he's an absolute gem of a human. Dave and I struck up a friendship immediately and he became the catalyst for me jumping feet first into the health and wellness space.

A Miraculous Meeting in Bolivia

My first segue into that world was in April 2021 when Dave, with contagious excitement, introduced me to Vladimir (Zev) Zelenko—a man who, in Dave's words, was, "Absolutely amazing, downright inspirational, and totally disrupting the treatment of COVID-19."

The day I met Zev in person for the first time in early August 2021, he had just discovered that his aggressive, rare, and terminal cancer had returned. From that point on, right through to his last days on this Earth, he possessed no fear of dying because he had divine faith that his higher power would take him to a better place, and was bolstered by the knowledge that when it was his time, it was his time.

Zev had just moved to Florida from New York. During this specific period of time, Zev was in the middle of his war with Andrew Cuomo, the Press, and the government. I remember when I met Zev and then Googled him—all I could find was negative press from *Vanity Fair* to the *New York Times*. That was my first introduction to how blatant censorship and media control was; they had perverted the story of a hero, making him sound like a lunatic and sham.

After making the sudden move from New York to Florida, Zev was looking to start a business. The purpose of his business would be to condense his Zelenko Protocol (using a combination of Vitamin C, Vitamin D, Quercetin, and Zinc to either prevent COVID-19 or if used in higher doses, to help treat early COVID-19) into a single, easy-to-use supplement.

Previously, Zev had open-sourced his protocol to the masses so that people could treat the early stages of COVID-19 in their own backyards. His aim was to help as many people as possible heal quickly, avoid hospitalization, and alleviate some of the fear the media was perpetuating in the larger public consciousness.

I perceived the risks in being involved with a person like Zev who was at once so polarizing and also so heroic. I knew I was walking into the belly of the beast by helping Zev start a business that would work to make accessible, over-the-counter products that directly go against the narrative of mainstream media and the government; products that help people without dependency on Pharma. Products that empower people. I didn't jump into business and partnership with Zev until I fully believed in him and the products.

Zev's mission challenged me to take the questions I'd asked earlier and turn them into action. I had already known that I was called to:

1. Create a measurably more healthy, loving, and free world.

2. Enlist as a warrior fighting for my kids and future grandchildren to live in a healthier, friendlier world than the one we've seen.

3. Do this in the community; working alongside other warriors like Zev, his family, Dave, and the team we have built.

The moment I said yes to working with Zev I had a moment of clarity. People sometimes refer to this as a message or a moment of enlightenment. Some people even hear voices that they identify with God or the universe. For me, this particular moment of *"hell yes"* changed the trajectory of my life.

I jumped into collaboration with Zev with both feet and, together with an excellent team, launched Zev's business - Z-Labs - on July 1 with explosive results.

I Will Fear No Evil

The world was hungry for hope and Zev was a beacon. He was uncompromising in his approach, using only the highest quality ingredients in his supplements. So many people gravitated to him and his brand. His courage and tenacity were inspiring. I watched how the darker times in his own life, particularly with his own health journey, reimbursed him the faith and resolve to shine the light on the path forward for us all.

Just before Zev passed, on June 30, 2022 - just one day after the first birthday of Z-Labs - he repeated the same thing to me and many of our mutual friends. "God might not be ready to see me just yet. He may be saying, 'that Zev, he still has more to do.' Either way, I am ready."

I have never seen such serenity; Zev was ready for the evil on this side of the grass, or the grace and glory on the other side. He was simply in a state of consciousness that was totally detached from his body. He was at peace. I remember one of the last things Zev said to me, which I also heard him say to many others during that last week of his life. Zev repeated a passage from Psalm 23:

> *Though I walk through the valley of the shadow of death, I will fear no evil: for thou art with me. Your rod and your staff comfort me.*

I watched a man, a husband, a father, and a dear friend give his everything, every day, not only to his family but also to this world. Zev was committed to his quest to inspire and create the good that we are striving for–that will change the world of medicine forever. Zev will forever be in my heart and I will draw on his memory, courage, and fighting spirit to help guide me forward.

This business we built of Zev's has taught and exposed me to a magnitude of experiences, both highly rewarding and highly challenging during its one-year journey thus far. Suddenly, I found myself reaching out to banks I have dealt with for years who were now abruptly refusing to work with me and to extend credit. The big law and accounting firms refused to work with me because I was suddenly "too radical" for them. Being associated with Zev and Z-Labs branded me overnight as an Anti-Vaxxer and Conspiracy Theorist. Society and my peers, many of whom I had worked with for years, were actively and publicly shaming me for trying to help people.

But, as the wise Mahatma Gandhi said: "First they ignore you, then they laugh at you, then they fight you, then you win." It all leads up to this moment; the moment we win.

The Moment We Win

I won't tell you any more about how our current health system is broken; you already know that it's broken, and the doctors contributing to this book will give you the full picture far more effectively than I can. You probably have your own examples from your life, or from your friends and family.

We all have our own stories of hospital negligence - of doctors who are more interested in the dollar sign you represent than in you as an individual - a Pharma industry born to make money and hone profits, drug manufacturers and drug wholesalers who hold their drugs and products ransom to achieve obscene profits. Furthermore, instead of using their profits to reinvest in technology companies to actually help people, Pharma buys up other companies that threaten to disrupt their monopolistic industry. They violently acquire companies that aim to bring their technologies to the world to help people. Often, Pharma shelves and essentially "kills" other companies' tech and products to solidify the monopoly in which their own substandard drugs and products are the "only" option.

So, in an industry that is about as corrupt as it comes, which spends billions of dollars to lobby the US government, and is allowed to create products while holding zero liability, what do we do? Let them hold onto this perpetual cycle of greed, power, and money?

Or, do we try to band together? Do we actually try to do something about it? When I gathered together The Wellness Company's Chief Medical Team for the first time, I said:

> *"I don't believe the government is going to help solve this healthcare crisis. Why would they? They have helped to create it, to perpetuate it. They are owned by Big Pharma's lobbying efforts. But I don't believe a non-profit will solve this crisis either, because they rely on other people's money and cannot achieve a scale large enough to make a difference. The only option to solve this is a well-run, transparent, for-profit entity with pure and noble intentions etched in stone. This entity will be navigated by the very doctors who haven't just 'claimed' they want change, but have shown through their actions that they cannot be bought or manipulated. These doctors will always put the patient first, even when it puts everything on the line. They will always stand up for what is right and will sacrifice everything to hold the line. They will not only stand up against governments and their own medical boards, but they will not compromise their integrity for anything, even when threatened. Let us find those doctors and create a new system."*

Together, my Chief Medical Team and I etched those words into our hearts and our company's vision, mission, and *culture*. Today, as I read those words, I still think of Zev; and I always will. Launching Z-Labs helped me understand that blowing a hole in the current corrupt medical system requires making money; we have to beat them at their own game, or at least play on their field. An impactful company absolutely does need to make money and, to be clear, that is not our driving factor, nor our focus. Our success is measured by the people we help and whose lives we extend and make healthier. Money is a by-product of the Good we're doing. Even more importantly, money becomes the leverage we have to enact real change and fight corruption at the highest levels.

Creating Medical Freedom with TWC

This book, as with all books, has gone through many title and subtitle changes, but one thing never changed: we determined that this would be a book about hope, not a post-mortem rehashing of all the bad things that have happened over the past few years and even decades. I'd share with you some of the other titles we considered, but that would ruin the surprise for the next few books we're working on right now. The subtitle was never really in question. We knew that it would involve the words "wellness revolution" or "medical freedom" and, ultimately, we decided that the subtitle would be "Standing Up For Medical Freedom" because the spirit of this manuscript is that you will read it and be empowered to take a stand. After reading it, you'll meet your new Wellness tribe at www.twc.health where we'll begin taking steps together, one at a time, until we become an unstoppable force for Good, together.

Here are the four core tenets that The Wellness Company will adhere to, although the different facets and iterations of these tenets will be vast.

1.Unbiased Education or "The Well." Members will receive solid, unbiased, science-backed data and education. You will have a place to learn, explore, and ask questions to our Chief Medical Team, who you'll learn about in this book. They're a Marvel superhero crew of some of the most highly-respected and honest action-takers in medical freedom. We commit to providing a place of trusted information where what you are reading is not anchored to a "left" or "right" agenda. Our motivation comes from an unbiased, factual place; we will remain in that place of humility and humanity, uncorrupted by politics. Our media department, called "The Well." is evolving into educational video content and documentaries on how to keep both our bodies and our planet healthier. We are already in pre-production for a series of yoga, fitness, and meditation videos. We are also committed to training healthcare providers through Medical Universities that will start online and eventually take place in physical locations through retreats, summits, and even semester-long courses. We're already in discussions with some Medical Institutions about bringing our methodologies to the next generation of medical leaders.

2. Quality Products, or "The Marketplace." Did you know that many "health" products cloak themselves as something "good for you", but when examined under a microscope, they are full of additives, fillers, and chemicals? As an example: The Wellness Company purchased what Amazon dubbed as a "hot deal" for Melatonin capsules. The manufacturer stated a cost of sixty capsules for only fifteen dollars. We purchased this product and tested it at our third-party facility, finding that the product was only 10 percent Melatonin and 90 percent brown rice flour. This product, like so many others we have examined, claimed to be something it wasn't. This is a common danger when shopping at unregulated and unchecked marketplaces. Our goal is to produce high-quality, third-party-tested, and trusted products at fair prices. Our Signature Series has been developed by our Chief Medical Team and we have already launched a Vitality Line, with more products continually being developed as the world and our company evolves. We're as ready as you are to patronize a new type of marketplace where products have been validated and proven to be high quality. Who has time to research every ingredient and brand of every supplement they take? One marketplace where you trust everything. Period.

For those of you sick of fast-fashion and the questionable activities and work arrangements surrounding it, we're also preparing a new fitness line consisting of high quality equipment and clothing you can feel good about purchasing. The Wellness Company marketplace is going to quickly include third-party products we've done the diligence to test for you and deliver at a fair price so that you can give your body what it needs and deserves. We are eager to collaborate with business owners who produce great health and wellness products; come and submit your products for our Chief Medical Board to review. If they meet our quality and good manufacturing standards, we will love to include your products in our marketplace.

3. Patient-First Medical Care, or "Virtual Healthcare." We've learned that not all medical professionals are committed to helping you and your family in your time of need. Apparently, the Hippocratic Oath covenant so many doctors committed to in medical school didn't apply during a pandemic; when patients needed providers most. You'll learn in this book that it's been decades since doctors stopped thinking for themselves; beholden to the direction and funding of the government, insurance companies, hospital corporations, and Pharma to provide guidance. Even more atrocious is how many doctors accept their codependency on corporations and no longer lose sleep over their loss of autonomy to practice medicine with integrity. The Wellness Company is changing that, starting by educating a group of doctors in our virtual health system before expanding into Virtual and, eventually, inpatient and medical university care. Above all, do not harm. Act with integrity and empathy. You, the patient, come before profit here at The Wellness Company. This starts by having an independent, sacred relationship with your doctor.

4. Wellness Pharmacies. The Wellness Pharmacy group will consist of both owned and franchised Pharmacies that will, again, put the patient first. You are not a number. It's not about script volume per day, it's about caring for each and every individual. We expect our Wellness Company pharmacists to be available to answer questions and make unbiased recommendations free from consideration to the bottom line.

Real talk: pharmaceutical products have a much higher margin than naturopathic or holistic products; the margins can be astronomical. In order to keep our business accountable for equally emphasizing holistic health, we are keeping pharmaceutical costs at an absolute minimum. Our team will not be incentivized to sell a pharmaceutical product over a naturopathic or holistic product. From a cultural perspective, this allows our entire company to focus on what's best for the patients.

Being Well, Doing Good

The Wellness Company also has an aggressive reinvestment plan that will allow the Wellness Company to fund these goals:

1. We will franchise up to one thousand independent Pharmacies across the USA. This will help us scale our buying power when purchasing pharmaceutical drugs but will also set the foundation for building out our Wellness Center Network.

We will strategically acquire Surgery and MRI centers that will serve to offer both inpatient and other clinical services.

We will continue to invest in technology to help better personalize your healthcare. Our goal is that one day you will belong not to an insurance company, but to a more affordable and even more ubiquitous Wellness Company ecosystem with membership to an integrated network of inpatient, outpatient, pharmacy, virtual, and health maintenance opportunities in every city.

We also pledge to give back to your communities. Unlike many companies who leverage their "giving pledges" for media acknowledgment, and who don't usually follow through, The Wellness Company will generously support several charities, including:

a) **Zelenko Freedom Foundation:** One of the last initiatives by Zev before he passed was to fulfill his legacy through the Zelenko Freedom Foundation. The foundation is driven by the mission to invest in innovative health technologies and treatments that Big Pharma would normally acquire, in order to shelf or extinguish because they have the power to empower and impact people towards health sovereignty, not pharma dependency. I have personally seen some of the immunotherapy technologies and treatments they are providing capital for and it's wildly inspiring.

b) **Together 4 Them:** When I met Dave on that fateful trip to Bolivia, my heart shattered when he told me about his work fighting the horrendous world of human trafficking. We have since partnered with another friend: UFC Champion Vitor Belfort, and his wife Joanna, who started the T4T mission when Vitor's sister was taken by traffickers and never rescued. The Wellness Company will provide transitional care and professional psychological support to victims recently rescued from trafficking. In order to heal and thrive, they need tremendous care and support in transitioning back into the world while avoiding slipping back into the cycle of trafficking.

c) **Children's Health Defense (CHD):** We agree with Robert F. Kennedy Jr., who says, "The greatest crisis that America faces today is the chronic disease epidemic in America's children." CHD's mission is to end childhood health epidemics by working aggressively to eliminate harmful exposures, hold those responsible accountable, and to establish safeguards to prevent future harm. We're proud to be in partnership with CHD to protect the next generation actively, starting right now.

My intention is that you will allow The Wellness Company to earn your trust. I'll start by personally introducing you to each member of our Chief Medical Board at the beginning of each of their chapters. I'll include a brief summary of their professional contributions as well as their intentions going forward both with The Wellness Company as well as, on a larger scale, to a broken system we are committed to reforming.

I hope you will join our movement and support what we are trying to build: a better system of health and wellness.

Foster Coulson
July 2022
twc.health

Dr. Heather Gessling

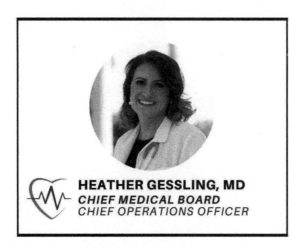

HEATHER GESSLING, MD
CHIEF MEDICAL BOARD
CHIEF OPERATIONS OFFICER

Heather Gessling is a warrior, a frontline general in the fight for better healthcare. As our Medical Board COO, she occupies the senior position in our medical operations and talks about how we can unite and stand together in our quest for proper, patient-led healthcare.

She has vast experience in running her own clinic and having escaped the world of corporate medicine, she has experienced and delivered firsthand the next wave of American healthcare.

Her Physician's Declaration, which she will tell you about, unified and united the sentiment of healthcare professionals across the nation. But that is not enough for her. She is not satisfied with mere words; she demands action institutionally, locally, and from patients themselves.

She is dogged and determined in her mission, making immense personal sacrifices as she jet-sets across the country spreading the word and demanding action. She has taken on the big guns and is continuing to do so. Her message is inspiring and I know that it will resonate with you on a deep intuitive level. Strap yourself in, it's quite the ride.

Foster Coulson

Chapter One

Finding Your Tribe

"When that which is difficult is overshadowed by the sense that you're doing the will of God; you're aligned with your purpose."

Zev Zelenko

I t was September 2021; the night before I was to fly to Puerto Rico for the first of many COVID-19 Summits. My husband and I remained seated at the dining room table after dinner and talked. My girls were sad I was leaving but distracted themselves by joyfully running around the house playing as my son, Evan, was washing the dishes. My husband was anxious about the traveling involved but he was glad Evan was joining me.

The air in the house felt heavy. Something was sitting especially heavy in my chest and it was making its way up my throat. It was hard to talk about what I knew was happening; what everyone knew was happening.

It was getting dark, so I turned on the lights of the chandelier over our heads and took in the warm gray hues from the walls. The pressure in my chest was building, and I simply had to spit out whatever was welling up inside of me.

After a deep breath, looking soberly and earnestly into my husband's eyes, I finally blurted out, "Honey, I'm being deployed. I've been called to duty. I'll need help with the kids. I am going to need your support."

That is one of the most memorable moments marking the life I have today.

As a doctor, I've always felt like a warrior, and this moment wasn't new to me. Over the past ten years, I traveled to a clinic in the town of Moberly, Missouri, forty-five minutes north of my hometown of Columbia because I knew it was my mission field. I knew it was where I was called to be.

I never stopped striving to do everything I could for my patients. I wanted to make their lives better. I wanted to make my hospital better. I wanted to be the best doctor possible at the same time as being the best mom and wife possible. I started a second practice in Columbia in 2019 to expand my reach. It was God's perfect timing that I did so because it allowed me to reach new patients before the horrors of COVID-19 hit in early 2020.

Between the two clinics, and with the collaborative relationships I had with three nurse practitioners and one physician assistant, I estimate my reach of care to have been approximately eight thousand patients.

Enlisting in the Fight

Unsurprisingly, in March 2020 my life underwent a dramatic shift. Although I've always been spiritually devoted to my practices, often spending the time driving from Columbia to Moberly praying earnestly for my patients and my hospital, it was at this moment that I experienced a true Awakening.

My colleagues Dr. McCullough and Dr. VanDeWater have expressed a similar feeling; our years of channeling our hearts into care for our patients suddenly and explosively evolved into an entirely different mission. Dr. VanDeWater will tell you in the next chapter about how she walked away from pharmacies to disrupt the pharmaceutical enterprise. Dr. McCullough surrendered every second of his free time to consistently and doggedly fight for truth. Dr. Amerling will tell you about how he sacrificed his comfortable life on the islands and the beautiful people in his community to fight for his principles.

And me? I also joined the fight for Truth and Life. I refused to follow orders from sources I didn't trust. I leaned in, dug into the research, and put my career on the line. I moved against the current of the mainstream flow, to truly figure out what was happening with this virus and how I could save patients. I relied on the Lord, as always, to guide me in my care for my patients and asked for His revelation of Truth.

He absolutely gave it.

Being responsible for several thousand patients in my Moberly and Columbia clinics, I eagerly sought the answer on how to save each and every life that walked through the doors.

The first enemy, indeed our greatest common enemy, was fear. I watched as fear often and repeatedly took hold of my patients' hearts and minds. Listening to the evening news, my patients were terrified. So many patients were obsessed with the information coming from their televisions.

I was desperate to do something to allay this fear. I consistently told my patients that listening to the news was ruining their health, encouraging practices that would damage them and ruin their mental health. I realized the importance of talking straight with my patients. I did not sugar-coat. They were coming to me for a reason. I armed them with recommendations on getting their Vitamin D levels to within the protective range against COVID-19 along with other beneficial supplements. I reassured them and told them to call me the first moment they got sick and we would start medications.

In truth, I was only scared for about two weeks. I too fell for the propaganda, but it didn't last long; once patients began getting sick I didn't have time to fear. I spent my time monitoring them closely via text and phone calls, and frequently checked in on their oxygen levels. I not only watched their pulse but I actively kept my finger on the pulse of new information that was being regularly released on how to manage COVID-19. Regimens were being tweaked and information was being shared between like-minded physicians online, similar to the physician support network we're now building with The Wellness Company.

Why Weren't they Curious?

The pandemic raged on, and in late 2020 my search for answers led me to understand ivermectin's effectiveness. Feeling satisfied with the vast benefits of using ivermectin in treating COVID-19 patients, I added it to my arsenal of medications.

At my hospital, I had been Chief of Staff for six years from 2015-2021, and Vice-Chief of Staff before that. During our monthly medical executive committee meetings, physician staff meetings, and interactions with peers online, I tried to point out the importance of these outpatient treatment modalities and the importance of nutrients in treating COVID-19.

And yet, although I had yet to see a single one of my patients die, many of my peers did not seem curious about the reasons for my success. They were essentially giving people cough medicine or acetaminophen and sending them home, telling patients there was nothing they could do. I have noticed for years that doctors easily gave scripts for azithromycin or other antibiotics for a viral cold. We've been inappropriately prescribing antibiotics for viral illnesses for decades.

Yet with COVID-19, perhaps due to additional public and media scrutiny, doctors put their hands up and would refuse to prescribe anything at all, much less what works. In addition, most physicians hid behind their specialties and would not join the fight to save patients. I know physicians of all specialties that stepped up to care for COVID-19 patients when their primary care colleagues failed to act. Dr. McCullough estimated last fall that there were perhaps five hundred physicians in the US willing to administer COVID-19 outpatient treatments or stand up for effective inpatient treatments—this includes refusing toxic medications. I am embarrassed for my peers. They failed their patients.

While my colleagues threw their hands up and, in some cases, wouldn't even consult with patients in person because of their own crippling fear of COVID-19, I begged them to see how many lives were being saved through safe, cheap, and widely available medications.

I broke COVID down for my peers, teaching them the different phases of the virus: Phase One, which lasts five to seven days, is the viral replication stage; Phase Two is the inflammo-thrombotic phase, which can be prolonged. I treated a mix of patients in the early infection stage as well as later on in the inflammatory phase. I had many people already in the inflammatory phase by the time they called me, and some who had already reached critical condition. For all cases, I used a combination of hydroxychloroquine or ivermectin, azithromycin (which is not only an antibiotic but also has anti-viral and anti-inflammatory properties,) or perhaps even stronger antibiotics and steroids.

I used many vitamins, oral and intravenous, and over-the-counter items such as famotidine, Benadryl, and melatonin, all for different reasons. I learned in 2021 to use stronger steroid doses if needed. It wasn't until mid-2021 that we learned we needed to increase the ivermectin dose. Nevertheless, nobody was dying—not a single patient of mine through to July 2021. I shared these results with my colleagues (and administrators) and it was like speaking to a brick wall. I will say it again, why were they not curious?

Despite feeling mostly alone in my efforts for the entire first year of the COVID-19 pandemic, I did have one local colleague for whom I am thankful: Dr. George Prica, who also understands the benefits of ivermectin and hydroxychloroquine. We were able to meet at a restaurant down the street from our respective clinics on a cold, wet day in December 2020 to discuss the wonders of these two medications—mostly regarding ivermectin.

He brought along some printouts, and I brought along a pre-med student. It was an energizing experience; it is critically important not to feel alone. This type of relationship is what it takes to save lives. There may have been only two or three more doctors in all of the mid-Missouri area that were prescribing it like we were. We had a local pharmacy that was on our side and did not deny the medication. We knew we were right about the medication. We looked at the mechanisms. We looked at the data. We had definitive observational experience proving that it was beneficial.

I knew it was going to be attacked because it worked. When the media "hit" pieces against ivermectin swamped the news in the late summer of 2021, I was completely unsurprised. I was only surprised that it did not happen sooner. The day we went to lunch happened to be my pre-med student's last day, and my parting words to her were, "Now you KNOW COVID."

When the Delta variant hit in the summer of 2021, it became obvious that patients weren't responding in the same ways to the arsenal, or "cocktail."

That July, I attended an America's Frontline Doctors event in San Antonio, Texas. Some of us had already interacted online or shared notes in common social media groups, but many of us hadn't yet met personally. It was at this event that I first met Dr. Ryan Cole and Dr. Richard Urso. Together, we enjoyed a sort of magical moment where the camaraderie was effortless. Our shared curiosity about the scientific aspects of COVID-19 led us to support one another with Delta and forge a powerful relationship that led to many educational summits across the country. It was invigorating to meet with even more clinicians who were deeply motivated to save lives with me, regardless of what hospital protocols or governmental agencies advised, or indeed failed to advise. We united our efforts to help build the tribe of warriors for the Truth regarding COVID-19.

The Importance of Nutritional Supplementation

When I learned about hydroxychloroquine early on in the pandemic, my entire perspective on medicine changed. I had already discovered through personal research that nutrients such as zinc, Vitamin C, and Vitamin D had a significant impact on the clinical outcome of COVID-19 infection. Research showed that chronic illnesses, such as diabetes, that led to zinc deficiencies were associated with poor outcomes. Like so many of my fellow doctors on the TWC Chief Medical Board, I came to understand that *it's all about the nutrients.*

(Side note–many patients that come to me have gone a bit overboard on zinc. Too much can lead to copper deficiency. Education is key regarding supplements.)

When I developed an understanding regarding the importance of nutrients, I was able to easily understand the mechanism of hydroxychloroquine. Simply put, hydroxychloroquine pulls zinc into the cell; zinc inhibits viral replication. In lay terms: the virus has trouble with replication when the body is sufficiently supplemented with zinc. Hydroxychloroquine and ivermectin loaded the gun, as the late Dr. Zelenko stated, but zinc pulled the trigger.

This was a revelation that may have saved millions of lives. It helped me save thousands. It helped my awakened peers save thousands more in their practices.

My friends, COVID-19 was treatable, and we treated it.

Reasons for Nutrient Deficiencies

In medical school, it was never conveyed to me how common of an issue nutrient deficiencies were. Thankfully, that wisdom has become more commonplace these days, although not as common as I'd like among my fellow physicians. However, when I was in medical school, my instructors actually belittled vitamins and supplements in general, suggesting that they were, at best, placebos, and at worst, a waste of time and money.

Nutrient deficiencies are common, especially among people with chronic illnesses and those who are taking medications. It wasn't until after medical school and residency that I understood this fact and the significance it had in impacting an individual's health.

To point out an example of the lack of understanding MDs have regarding deficiencies, there was a long post that a local physician published stating why nutrient deficiencies are not really a problem. In it, he falsely stated that essentially everyone receives sufficient nutrients in a typical American diet.

This highlights to me what a sad state of affairs the medical community is in. It's also worth noting that his post was created soon after a post I released regarding the necessity of Vitamin D for COVID-19 prevention and treatment was spread to my local community, and this type of counter-post was not an isolated event. It begs the question: why were physicians so against utilizing vitamins?

The second reason for the widespread national issue with deficiencies is low nutrient levels in our food. Our foods are depleted because our soil is depleted. We are only receiving a fraction of the nutrients that we would perhaps have received thirty or forty years ago. This is not hard to research and I encourage you to do so. I won't get into what got us to this point, but it's no wonder that once an individual becomes awakened to the state of our food supply, self-reliance through gardening and growing our own food shortly follows.

I do believe organics are best. I understand how hard it can be to keep organic foods in supply at home, but there's a strong case to be made for simply making this happen, even if that involves organic meal delivery versus growing your own food. Organic foods aren't merely (theoretically) more likely to be free from pesticides, herbicides, GMOs, and fertilizers, but they've been shown to be higher in nutrients, polyphenols, antioxidants, Vitamin C, beta-carotene, Vitamin A, protein, and nitrates–among many other benefits. They also contain essential digestive enzymes which help our body absorb nutrients.

At TWC, we have formulated a suite of supplements that are created, designed, and approved by MDs, PharmDs, and NDs. They use natural ingredients from trusted sources and are backed by medical studies. We know and understand the importance of essential nutrients. We visualize a world that relies more on preventative care of our bodies so that we can utilize nutraceuticals before resorting to pharmaceuticals. Prevention over treatment.

What boggles my mind about medical school and residency is the complete absence of education about nutritional health. This is crucial for effective and efficient cellular function, including immune function. We plan to change that at TWC. We have big plans.

Family Bravery

From the very beginning of the pandemic, when hydroxychloroquine was attacked in the media to when ivermectin was labeled a "horse dewormer" in the late summer of 2021, it was always clear to me what I was up against. It was easy to recognize the propaganda designed to clear the field for a concerted push to coerce the public to willingly, and unwillingly, take part in an investigational gene based therapy treatment that has, to date, caused incalculable harm both those who complied as well as those who have been persecuted for exercising caution, skepticism, and medical freedom.

Although my awakened colleagues and I were experiencing tremendous success in treating patients, President Trump's original praise of hydroxychloroquine and other early treatment measures soon turned towards a race for a vaccine. The governmental guidance on actually treating COVID-19 in the outpatient setting was basically to do nothing.

By April 2021, the realization dawned on me that I had gone over a year with no patient deaths, but I didn't stop and celebrate; I was too busy keeping my head down and keeping people alive.

It was a different story for many of my colleagues, as the mainstream news that COVID-19 was a deadly and untreatable virus had gotten to their heads. Between their patients who were dissatisfied with ineffective care and those within my clinics, I had no shortage of cases to treat. I remained determined, though, and never let the mainstream fears affect the way I treated patients.

It was about that time that I explained to my kids that it wasn't just my job to keep them safe, but that God had also given me the charge of helping save His children all over the country. My husband was a wonderful help, and he knew the support I needed. At times, the response from my family was solemn; they understood people were scared and that my job was to keep them safe and well. They had gotten used to me constantly caring for patients that were already mine or that had come to me because no one else would take care of them. On the odd occasion, my children were frustrated and sad because I had to travel to COVID-19 summits as well as many other efforts to bring truth, which included traveling to D.C. to speak with senators, going to different state legislatures, or attending the March Against the Mandates Rally in D.C. Throughout these events, my husband cheerfully and faithfully held down the fort. He offered to help with editing for different tasks involved with the summits. He drove me back and forth to the airport when needed. He did not complain when I had to be gone. A soldier can not do it alone.

A fellow soldier in the fight during this time of war has been my seventeen-year-old son. My son is fully aware of the battle for truth happening around us. His diplomatic skills and "all hands on deck" attitude have allowed him to serve in numerous ways. He has helped me and my colleagues diligently in any way he can including prayer or chauffeuring us around when needed.

Even this morning, he stepped away from his busy life to text me and provide me with advice for my writing time. My son isn't afraid to work hard for his beliefs and his country, and he has not been afraid to fight for the truth at his school. He fought diligently against the continued use of masks, discouraged his peers from injecting themselves with experimental products, and he provided information to his peers regarding the importance of nutrition. He will soon be the youth pastor intern at our local church. In so many ways, while surrounded by so many bad actors, my brave son embodies hope for the next generation. He is exceedingly, beautifully, and totally brave.

The Physician's Declaration of Independence

So much was born out of the America's Frontline Doctor's Conference of July 2021. In particular, Dr. Richard Urso gave a presentation about COVID-19, revealing what was working in his practice. I listened intently, picking up on the similarities between our methods of treatment, and at the conclusion of his talk, I found myself dashing up to him after the presentation.

"Dr. Urso," I said, "everything you said you're doing I'm doing as well, but things are changing. It's not working like it used to."

"You are right. I know. We have to change something." He calmly replied.

I told him I had just got off the line with one of my nurses before his lecture, and I had told her to increase a patient's dose of ivermectin and do it daily for six days instead of every other day like we all had been doing.

"That is what I just did with a patient as well. We have to increase the ivermectin."

Later in the conference, Dr. Urso shared with me that he was starting the Pandemic Health Alliance, now called the Global Covid Summit, having evolved from an organization of doctors surviving the pandemic together to an organization focused on hosting summits. A short time later, I found myself in Puerto Rico with Dr. Urso, Dr. Ryan Cole, Dr. Brian Tyson, Dr. John Littell, Dr. Robert Malone, Dr. Mark McDonald, and Dr. Pierre Kory. While there, we grouped around a large table and collaboratively edited a document that my friend (and former college roommate) Saundra Traywick, Dr. Littell, and I had initially drafted for a Physician's "Declaration of Independence," including a declaration of patient-physician autonomy. There have now been thousands of signatures from physicians and medical professionals on that Declaration.

The most important concerns and covenants among my awakened medical peers and I can be summarized with these three topics:

1. The autonomy of the physician-patient relationship is sacred.

2. The dangers of the COVID-19 experimental gene therapy treatment, called a "vaccine," are scientific, not opinion-based. Although multiple governmental and mainstream agencies and organizations are not highlighting that message (and labeling it as disinformation), we signers of the Declaration are committed to holding the line and supporting patients who stand for truth and medical freedom.

3. Early outpatient treatment is key. Telling people to wait at home helplessly until they are in a critical enough condition to enter a hospital is cruel, unnecessary, and potentially homicidal.

Today I'm saddened, maybe even righteously angry, that the bravery of many of those doctors signing the Declaration seemed to dry up with the ink.

Where are they? The Declaration is only powerful if we take action. Problem is, I honestly don't think those doctors were given the tools to implement change. We can't just preach to the choir, blowing more hot air into the environment. We have to take intelligent, resourceful action against our enemies.

Here at TWC, *we're putting our money where our mouth is;* we're fighting corrupt organizations in government and healthcare with their game; we're leveling up to create a critical mass resistance of Americans (and eventually global citizens) who reject everything corporate healthcare related. We're going to get them where it hurts, in their pocketbooks.

They don't care about our cries. They don't care about skyrocketing death rates. They don't care about the truth.

That's why I joined TWC and left the other organizations. That's why, Dr. Richard Amerling and I, who had been working on forming a telehealth company, were introduced to Foster and heard his vision for The Wellness Company, we immediately jumped on board. Other organizations approaching the telehealth niche have struggled to keep patient costs low, struggled to enlist and retain doctors, and struggled to keep their intentions pure and the finances transparent. Worse yet, countless organizations don't *do* anything; they just talk about doing.

I don't want to just organize another self-congratulatory summit providing a reunion for the Freedom Fighters. These events are uplifting to those fighting the fight, but I want to participate in driving millions of people towards freedom through telemedicine unadulterated by greedy corporations, independent Wellness Pharmacies uncontrolled by insurance, nutraceuticals that don't kill our health, as well as education that empowers us to march around Big Pharma until their walls crumble.

What we all need to understand is that the way we have chosen to fight for the last two years has thus far failed to stop governmental overreach or prevent children from receiving the experimental gene therapy that is falsely called a vaccine. It hasn't stopped pharmaceutical companies from exploiting the citizens of this country or big corporations from demanding employees to accept a medical intervention for the "good of humanity"; one that provides no societal benefit.

Unfortunately, even the Freedom Fighters have their flaws. I was bullied and defamed when I chose to join TWC. Members of the organization that I had started the fight for the truth with and individuals that support it made astoundingly inflammatory statements about me for choosing to pursue this opportunity to enact real change. I've never had anything like it happen in my life. I felt like my family had turned on me.

In my heart, I love all my fellow freedom fighters and I trust that many, if not most of us, will wind up, again, in a restored tribe through God's grace and forgiveness. I'm presently disheartened that so many chose to disenfranchise a fellow warrior after that warrior fought so hard and unselfishly alongside them. It frustrates me further when you consider the obvious fact that there are not enough soldiers in the fight to begin with. Indeed, the most painful part is to know that we are already outnumbered. There's no time nor resources for petty dissension among the ranks.

I thanked the Lord daily, though, for His divine protection and amazing providence in bringing me into such an ideal new company. The song *Reckless Love* by Cory Asbury became my mantra during this time. The words of the song - "You have been so, so good to me" - kept me going every day through the heartache as well as the daily new adventures of building this company and at the same time growing my amazing Direct Primary Care clinic, Gessling Family Wellness.

My friends Dr. VanDeWater and Dr. Schmidt, who you will read about later, have similar stories. The warriors have been bruised by colleagues they trusted like family. With grace, I attribute the emergence of negativity and even maliciousness in others to battle fatigue among good but otherwise weary soldiers. Sometimes old habits or previously suppressed character flaws resurface under the weight of fatigue. There has been so much stress fighting the "system" that along the way there are inevitable and hurtful events that have taken place.

I have a feeling you might like me to elaborate on all those events, but unfortunately, that may prevent future reconciliation. I believe the way back to harmony happens from believing the motives and hearts of those standing up for truth. The lesson is that we have to protect our own. Egos have to go. I hope and pray that as we start coming out on the other side that reconciliation will happen and we can all join forces to fight together again as we win the war.

A friend of mine who runs a large team of powerful truth-speaking influencers reminds her staff at every meeting, "We are each strong alone, but together we are stronger. The only way out is through, but the best way through is together. When we're united, each one of us is infinitely more impactful."

"I Trust My Doctor Less Than Anybody"

My friend, Saundra Traywick, whom I mentioned earlier as a key contributor to the Declaration, is an example of the disempowerment that parents feel within the medical community ecosystem.

Saundra, a successful interior designer and businesswoman whose daughter acquired PANDAS (Pediatric Autoimmune Neuropsychiatric Disorders Associated with Streptococcal Infections) from a strep infection, has gone through an awakening over the past several years. I am immensely thankful for her; she helped bring me to the point where I recognized lies and inadequacies in my medical education.

Like almost anybody who takes the time to research and dig into mainstream medicine, nutrition, pharmaceuticals, and the insurance company stranglehold on physicians and pharmacies, Saundra lost faith in the medical community when her daughter was diagnosed in 2014. Saundra found herself in the position of so many magnanimous and loving parents who have sick children and cannot get answers from the medical community. It was her who realized what was making her daughter very sick. Because of Saundra's tenacity, her daughter was able to be treated and have a near-full recovery relatively quickly.

Since then, she continues to seek truth for a vast number of medical conditions that doctors simply will not acknowledge. She reads blogs and articles, talks to other parents, and avidly seeks information in every corner of the internet that will help her family. Because of this experience, she learned that donkey milk has amazing immunity-promoting properties, so she and her husband left their well-established jobs and life, bought a farm with donkeys, and are now suppliers of donkey milk.

Once Saundra began posting things she had uncovered online, I was disturbed and bothered by what ensued. Although Saundra posted about things that were empirically verifiable, she also posted things that she, as a mother with a horrible medical experience, had every right to express. And if you know anything about Mama Bear energy, you know that it's a force to be reckoned with.

I was in shock when my physician peers on social media wrote dismissive and derogatory replies to Saundra's posts that told of her experience and her distrust of medical professionals. At that moment, I lost a lot of respect for my profession. I saw them berate, belittle, and denigrate somebody publicly, using their "medical authority" as an excuse to be bullies. Any medical professional with an open mind would embrace Saundra and encourage her to keep asking questions, to keep evolving as her and her daughter's medical advocate, and to continue sharing her revelations. They would allow her to continue her healing through sharing, and to keep seeking community.

These medical professionals made a public disgrace of themselves and our profession. I'll share with you the answer to a question you may have asked before: Do doctors have big egos?

Yes. It is disturbingly common. Among so many of my colleagues (not the ones in this book, of course,) their education becomes an idol; their MD or DO degree becomes their license to close out any lay person's research or opinions.

Only recently, I had a local nephrologist tell me that I would never be able to convince him to "turn his back on mainstream medical science." They are deeply entrenched and engulfed in their titles and connection to mainstream medical science. This is the perfect stage for disaster for their patients.

Do you want to know how Dr. Vladimir Zelenko came across his revolutionary findings concerning the use of a zinc ionophore to treat COVID-19? The same way my friend Saundra did. He got online and performed internet research, internet research that started with an open mind. Zev's research has saved hundreds of thousands, perhaps even millions of lives around the world.

I recall a conversation I had a few years ago with a dermatologist friend of mine who sent his adult daughter to me as a patient. She was highly educated about her condition. She knew more about her endocrine condition than maybe even I knew about it. She was, in fact, teaching me things I hadn't previously known.

She apologized to me, saying "I know I can really throw out a lot of information."

I replied that I was appreciative of our conversations and that I always enjoy learning from patients. I believe that her father was both surprised and happy to hear this. Perhaps it is because this mentality is not common among physicians. I wish more patients were like her; well-researched, self-advocates who take full responsibility for their own health, and I wish more physicians were willing to learn from their patients.

What Being Brave Means

Brave means paying attention to patients and the parents of patients. I am not just broadcasting this message to my physician peers, but to society in general. I feel nauseated when I replay scenes in my mind of parents coming in to talk to me about childhood vaccines and dismissing their valid concerns. I admit my prior ignorance on the subject. I regurgitated what little I was taught but, my goodness, was there more that I needed to learn.

I do not know exactly why there is an explosion in autism. I do not know exactly why there is an explosion in ADHD. I do know that every parent has the right to question traditional medicine until it is able to give answers to the explosion of chronic diseases in children. Is it due to the prevalence of toxic food? Is it due to the dramatic increase in the number of childhood vaccines? I don't know. Why is this not an emergency?

Pediatrician Dr. Paul Thomas performed a thorough and comprehensive analysis comparing vaccinated children to unvaccinated children in his practice, and the results came through loud and clear: his unvaccinated patients did not have anywhere near the levels of chronic illness or even acute infections that his vaccinated pediatric patients had. This analysis is not isolated.

Being brave means ignoring the roar - The roar may be from family, friends, social media, mainstream media, alternative media, education, entertainment, work policies, politicians, or advertising. The roar may consist of fear, propaganda, charm, distraction, or deception. How do you ignore the roar?

Brave means defining the lies - Do governmental agencies and the Biopharmaceutical Complex have unblemished reputations? Nope. Ok, do they even have good reputations? Nope. All it takes is a quick search of lawsuits against pharmaceutical companies to see how untrustworthy they are.

Recently, CDC Director Rochelle Walensky admitted that they "stumbled" in their "big moment" and has outlined plans to revamp the CDC. So why are we as a society placing so much blind faith in these entities?

It has become a cult.

In addition, spokespeople for certain three letter agencies became adored personas equivalent to saints or gods. I have said before that parents have unfortunately trusted their children to the gods of Pfizer and "Science" (the new science that says it is ok to inject children with experimental substances). How does this happen?

The good news is that I have noticed more and more parents coming into my clinic stating that, due to their mistrust of pharmaceutical companies and recommendations from governmental agencies, they no longer want to vaccinate their children. Not only that, they are disturbed by what they had previously allowed their children to be injected with and that they wish they could turn back time.

I tweeted this observation and there was an immense outpouring of consensus among parents across the country, and even further afield. At the time of writing, that simple post has garnered twenty thousand likes, over six thousand retweets, as well as over a thousand comments from parents stating that their trust is gone and they are done. One of the comments even called it the Post of the Century. The statement clearly resonated with parents.

Brave means taking back your rightful position as lion or lioness of your family -
There must be a realization that the responsibility for yourself and your
children lies with you. Not the government, not your pediatrician, not
your family physician. You. Take it back. Stand up for your autonomy.

I look back to when my youngest child was born in 2016. I remember
going back and forth in my mind about the decision to give her the
Hepatitis B vaccine in the hospital. I was at the beginning of my journey
in waking up to the overreach of medicine. As a physician, I was genuinely
worried about what the nurses would think of me, what my peers taking
care of me in the hospital would think of me, and what declining the
vaccine meant for me as a physician. My daughter, as did all my other
children, received that vaccine at birth. Shame on me, though. If I saw
no need for my newborn to get a Hep B vaccine a day into her precious,
perfect life for a disease that she had zero risk of contracting, why did I
allow myself to let them give it to her?

I am shocked and saddened, taken aback by the inhumanity of what
physicians have done to parents. It is tragic. If I, as a physician, could not
say no to what I deemed unnecessary then how do I expect non-clinical
parents to have the fortitude to say no?

Yet many *have* said no and I applaud them. This is not about the
vaccine debate. My point is that parents need to be able to be safe in the
medical system to navigate it their own way. It is time for a paradigm
shift. Parents are ultimately responsible for their children; they will
be the ones caring for their children should an injury from a medical
intervention occur and they should not have to make decisions out
of fear of retaliation by the medical community or pressure from the
medical community.

Here at TWC, we are committed to restoring the sacredness of the
patient-doctor relationship, restoring patient autonomy and involvement
in their care. Dr. Richard Amerling will share with you in a later chapter
more technical and shocking reasons for which the physician-patient
relationship has deteriorated. In the meantime, let's ponder why people
are right to distrust their doctors.

I, as a physician, honor you. I am proud of you for taking personal responsibility for your health and the decisions you make for your body. You are right to suspect that your doctor is following protocols that are not in your best interest. You are right to be wary of insurance and pharmaceutical company kickbacks. You are right to want something better. That's why you're reading this book.

The Anatomy of Physician-Patient Distrust

There are two easily identifiable primary reasons for which patients are becoming increasingly wary of their physicians—even, as is the case in some cases, scared to enter a hospital or doctor's office.

Compassionate and trustworthy care seems to have disappeared. The onus isn't just on the physicians who have lost their moral compasses. It's also on us patients to demand a higher standard of care. My colleagues and I here at TWC aim to support the movement to demand a higher level of care. You must express your wishes to your doctors. I cannot guarantee they'll be met with compassion or even respect, but every stitch we sew into the resistance to medical tyranny is a step in the direction of freedom.

1) The autonomy of the patient-physician relationship.

Autonomy in the patient-physician relationship implies that patients receive information about their diagnosis, treatment, and prognosis that empowers the patient to make informed decisions. In an autonomous patient-physician relationship, patients are involved in decisions in a two-way dialogue about what treatments or medications they feel are best for them. As you'll see described in Dr. VanDeWater's chapter, insurance companies have entirely too much control over the care of patients. What we experienced with caring for COVID-19 patients is that pharmacists stood in the way of patients receiving the life-saving medications they needed. As

Dr. McCullough described in the first chapter, sometimes doctors willingly prescribe treatments that aren't in the best interest of the patient because the doctors are following a corporate protocol, not their personal convictions. These are two among many examples of the deterioration of the sacred patient-physician relationship, which will be further discussed in Dr. Richard Amerling's chapter later in this book.

2) Doctors may not be open to learning new things or may be resistant to following a line of thinking that may be different from what they have been originally taught.

As you saw with my friend Saundra, not every doctor is open to listening to patients, even when the patient has done more digging on a condition than a doctor. This problem stems from ego, pride, defensiveness, laziness, a God-complex, and perhaps a myriad of other economic or psychological factors.

Over the past several decades, authorities have taken away the physician's ability to make decisions *for* the patients. When I was in school I learned Evidence-Based Medicine (EBM) theory. EBM is essentially a practice in which clinicians recommend standard treatments without consideration of a patient's lifestyle, relationships, habits, and other key factors related to illness. When I learned of EBM, I was horrified; I immediately rejected a practice that takes away the individuality of the patient and creativity in developing a treatment plan that is in the best interest of the patient. My colleague, Dr. Richard Amerling, will dive deeper into this in Chapter Seven. It's a doozy, so hold onto your hats.

Among the reasons EBM practices exist are these:

1. Hospital employees are owned by a corporation, the business that is the hospital. Often, the business makes decisions and recommendations for the doctor, as opposed to the other way around. Yes, it's as terrifying as it sounds.

2. Independent practices have become few and far between. The margins from insurance reimbursements are too low and the costs associated with taking insurance are too high. I preface this by saying that Direct Primary Care clinics are opening across the country like wildfire but there are still not enough independent practices. It is too expensive to take insurance. It takes multiple employees to push through billing for insurance claims and manage them. Because of this, many physicians have sold out to hospitals.

3. As Dr. Amerling and Dr. VanDeWater illustrate in this book, hospital environments are focused on achieving "quality numbers" and Key Performance Indicators, not on practicing true medicine and healing patients.

4. Like the micromanaging Dr. VanDeWater illustrates in Chapter Three, doctors are under pressure to keep the administration happy and not "rock the boat".

5. Insurance companies are pushing various benchmarks that have little to do with patient care and this diverts the focus a physician should have on a patient. They are already pushed to see more and more patients. Today, the landscape is even more dire direr; the CDC and NIH have been giving recommendations for care; even the White House feels as though they have the right to prescribe care with broad, over-generalized statements and mandates. Your doctor's office visits are largely dictated by benchmarks and numbers coming top-down from impersonal organizations that know nothing about you, your body, or your psyche. When a doctor is checking off boxes on a computer-generated questionnaire, he or she may not find the time nor freedom to ask you about things that truly matter, such as your interpersonal relationships, your diet, or other critical factors to health.

Doctors have a fiduciary responsibility to patients that's been lost. From the moment I finished my residency, I focused on my patients and relied on God's guidance and provision as well as my own efforts to learn real medicine. By bringing my covenant with God into my covenant with my patients, I have been more open-minded, humble, and passionate about seeing the truth.

If the medical community does not change, we simply won't make medical advances and improvements. When the doctor becomes robotic and when EBM is applied, physicians no longer fight to observe and improve things. They are little more than highly-educated order takers. Medicine isn't improved top-down. Boots on the ground experience and observations helped save lives but it could have been more.

The Future of Independent Practices

In May 2021, I felt with the utmost clarity that the Lord was telling me I would be leaving both of my practices and starting a Direct Primary Clinic.

My initial reaction was that this was crazy. How could I pull that off?

However, I knew that all of the issues that I have highlighted were happening in my clinics or were going to be getting worse. I feared the investigational gene-based therapy called a "vaccine" for COVID-19 would be mandated. I also despised being in clinics that insisted I wear a mask despite the harm they caused. I knew I needed more time with my patients and more control over my practice.

In June, I decided to submit a hand in my ninety-day notice that I would be leaving at my Columbia practice. I didn't know what would happen with my Moberly practice, but later that decision was made for me.

At the beginning of August, I was asked by my CEO in Moberly to step down from my position as Chief of Staff due to my publicly posted concerns about the "vaccine". He said, "We just can't have that."

Next, I was told to either obtain the investigational gene-based therapy, otherwise known as "the jab," or submit to weekly testing. I declined both options and. I was terminated.

I knew what I had to do next. Within two weeks I had opened up Gessling Family Wellness, a Direct Primary Care clinic. This type of clinic is opening up everywhere. It is not complicated and I have helped many colleagues make the switch. Often, they express their disbelief that they did not walk away from the "system" sooner.

There are no constraints on insurance. Most of these clinics, including mine, are membership based. I have very little time constraints with patients now. I can care for my patients in more flexible ways, and insurance claims are no longer involved with visits, which changes things completely. Most physicians are pressured by their employers to squeeze more and more patients into their day in order to increase their margin as insurance companies are paying less and less. Direct Primary Care, or cash-based practices, are the best way to eliminate the influences of insurance companies and the pressures of hospital-based practices.

An additional point to be made is the extraordinary increase in the number and salaries of hospital administrators over the last several decades. Who is feeding those salaries? Why are so many administrators necessary? Could it be unnecessary governmental regulations?

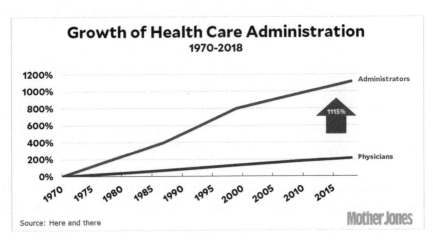

Solutions for The Reader

My earnest request is that you consider a few practical steps for your health, and for the health of future generations.

When possible, I implore you to speak openly to your doctor about what you need. Just this week one of my friends took her son for a well-care visit. The doctor asked one of a list of questions on her iPad and the mother took the time to stop and say, "Doctor, I'm worried about my son's psychological health. I'm scared that if he continues with this behavior, he'll have a lot of problems socializing next school year, and perhaps forever."

This independent doctor (i.e. not aligned with a hospital) invested 45 minutes pouring wisdom and love into my friend and her child. She did not prescribe medication in order to quickly end the visit and move on to the next patient, and my friend was immensely grateful for this. When she left, she immediately took the doctor's compassionately given advice and made demonstrable changes to her parenting, setting new boundaries and expectations for the child.

She wrote to the doctor the next day, saying, Dr., my child is like a different person. He slept better last night than he has in over a year. It was so hard for me to set boundaries and expectations, but after initially disrespecting and shrugging me off, he took me quite seriously when I created consequences for his insolence. I feel empowered and in control for the first time in seven years.

This is what happens when a doctor has more time. The amount of true change that encounter created is extensive. Did it save multiple counselor visits or other physician visits? Did it possibly change the child's entire life? This is real medicine. This is the way I practice. I hope to provide care that reduces healthcare costs as well as reduce the need for pharmaceutical intervention.

Talk to your doctor. Find an independent physician who is going to give you the time of day. Allow that doctor to be a trusted, respected source of wisdom and information. And if your doctor isn't going to respect you and your family, we anticipate that TWC can help you.

The only way we restore the sacredness of the physician-patient relationship is to demand it. The patients must insist on leaving practices that don't educate nor respect them. If patients don't migrate, things won't change.

Dr. Peter McCullough is more bearish on this migration than I. He wants us to express ourselves but stay with our doctors. I understand and respect that, but there also comes a point where we have to look out for our family's health and if your doctor is practicing on a foundation of lies, you cannot continue to support that practice. When hospitals see that their patients are unsatisfied (thereby threatening their bottom lines), they'll be forced to shift, to change, and to listen. I hear daily from patients that they want to do everything they possibly can to avoid having to not ever set foot in a hospital again. They have lost all trust.

I suspect that we have to make it hurt for these tyrannical corporate entities because they're not going to have a "come to Jesus" moment unless it shows up in their pocketbooks. TWC is here to provide access to truth. We're here to provide support for nutraceutical supplementation before resorting to pharmaceuticals that are being over-prescribed in overwhelming numbers of patients.

Finally, I encourage you to find your health tribe. I know a friend who fasts on Sundays with a local pastor in his community. When asked why he fasts on Sundays, he stated, "I have raised two children, but now I am raising the consciousness of the entire world." In that moment I located the precise spirit of The Wellness Company and the communities you and I lead from coast to coast, including right in the middle of the country where I am. We're all on the same team.

Through TWC, you'll connect with countless doctors as well as healthy-minded lay people at www.twc.health, but don't stop blessing your local community and reaching across religious or political party lines to hold hands and hold the line.

As Chief Operating Officer of The Wellness Company Medical Board, I commit to serving as a general in this war; coordinating, supporting, and advising our physicians so that we can all bring medical freedom to your family. We are here to protect life amidst this culture of death. We are surrounded by attacks against life whether it be the censoring of life-saving information regarding early outpatient treatment for COVID or attacks on naturalistic ways of living. We are here to bring truth in the darkness and we're honored to have you in our ranks.

Welcome to the tribe.

Dr. Heather Gessling

Chapter One Takeaways

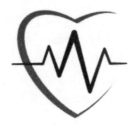

How do you feel? Inspired, awake, energized? Do you feel inspired to take action and join the fight, becoming another paragon of wellness? As Dr. Gessling so eloquently states, it is not enough to simply talk the talk, we must walk the walk. We have to take accountability and form a tribe, with a message and an identity that simply cannot be denied or refuted.

We are committed to a healthcare revolution, and we don't care whose toes we tread on to make that happen. We will take on the big guns, we will attack their bottom line, and as Dr. Gessling says, we will connect with patients on a human, individual level.

Dr. Gessling explains that what we put in our bodies is crucial to our health. Nutrition is crucial to not only maintaining a healthy lifestyle but in staving off critical illnesses before they have the opportunity to develop and grow. This is not an attitude that is widely accepted across the medical industry because supplements and food cannot be prescribed.

So, as Dr. Gessling suggests, come alongside www.twc.health and see if there is a tribe or a connection waiting for you. See if there is someone who can help and advise you on the best way to boost your health without damaging your body. I doubt you will be disappointed.

Foster Coulson

Dr. Peter McCullough

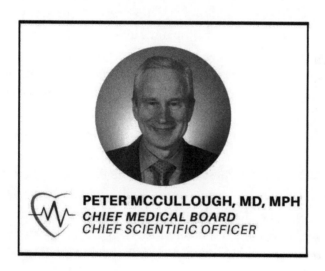

PETER MCCULLOUGH, MD, MPH
CHIEF MEDICAL BOARD
CHIEF SCIENTIFIC OFFICER

Dr. Peter McCullough brings a formidable reputation and relentless energy for the cause of medical freedom to The Wellness Company. His meteoric rise to the top as an academic internist and cardiologist came at an extremely young age, but he hasn't stopped there as he has become one of the most prominent physicians in America.

Dr. McCullough is trusted and respected in both the professional medical as well as layperson communities, being the most published person in the world in his field - the interface between heart and kidney disease - in history. Dr. McCullough has reached the highest stature of academic medicine, lecturing before the US FDA, the European Medical

Association Agency, and the New York Academy of Sciences. He was the main presenter at a US Congressional oversight panel for the FDA on a major product label expansion. He has dozens of peer-reviewed publications on the pandemic, particularly with regards to the treatment of the infection, over seven hundred and seventy overall publications in The National Library of Medicine, plus an additional one thousand-plus overall medical communications. He's served on two dozen data safety monitoring boards for large pharmaceutical, device, and in vitro diagnostic studies.

Dr. McCullough's addition to the team represents something significant for the Wellness Company. He is a well-known public figure regularly appearing on TV to advise against the dangers of a healthcare system that does not work for the benefit of the patient, but for the Biopharmaceutical Complex. When Dr. McCullough isn't seeing patients; he's writing articles, researching, testifying, or appearing on podcasts and news shows to provide accessible education even to non-academic audiences.

Dr. McCullough is chest-deep in the fight against the Complex, a fight which has seen him active in the courts, with his cases setting legal precedents that have led to multiple legal wins against a form that has, up to now, run rampant and unchecked.

Dr. Peter came to us through Dr. Richard Amerling, with whom he's been friends for over twenty years. He says that all the credit for bringing Dr. Peter to The Wellness Company lies with Dr. Amerling, citing brilliant synergy with our senior executive team from the first time we all met together in Florida. Following that meeting, he stated, "I have absolutely no doubt I have made the right choice. The Wellness Company is the place to be."

Foster Coulson

Chapter Two

Preparing Your Heart for The Next Wave

"A lot of life is about trying to turn bad experiences into something good. Usually if you work at it, you can figure out a way to do it. Even our worst misfortunes are gifts."

Robert F. Kennedy, Jr.

R obert F. Kennedy Jr. (affectionately known as "Bobby") once shared a story that forever defined my perception of what it means to be brave. As children, the Kennedys were told that there was no greater honor they could have in the course of their lives than to be alive during a time of great controversy; to play a role in the resolution and closure of a crisis. Today, we are at the tip of the spear; this is the 1776 moment of our lives.

Bobby has a fixed place as one of my heroes, and one of three heroes I'll reference in this chapter; a chapter designed to teach you how to prepare your heart and your spirit for the Next Wave.

He has modeled bravery in his advocacy for children through Children's Health Defense, and he has never been shy about boldly speaking aloud his convictions. What's more, Bobby has modeled relentless drive, tireless effort, and sincere appreciation for the work he has carved out the opportunity to do. My intention is that we all carry ourselves with that degree of grace and purpose. It is for that reason that my intention is not merely to tell you what bravery means, but to show you bravery throughout this chapter and through examples in my own life.

Rule Number One: bravery doesn't play well with complainers, victims, or those who feel entitled. Rather than approaching the long road to medical freedom ahead of us as some insurmountable task or burden, I invite you to embrace the message young Bobby heard growing up, which has inspired and led him to become one of the most important medical freedom fighters in history. This is our crisis moment; a moment during which we were born to contribute; something that won't be easy, but will bring us together in joy and appreciation for one another - our fellow medical freedom fighters.

To be alive at this time of great worldwide controversy, I propose, is our destiny. And now that we've survived the past few years of a particularly terrifying initiation into a world we didn't choose to live in, I invite you to join me in restoring the world to its rightful axis. This is your moment to live - and perhaps even cease to live - with honor.

In this chapter, I'll share the details and characteristics of three heroes in the recent global chaos alongside those of three villains, providing strategies on how to defeat them and help others along the way.

I'm personally intoxicated with the honor of helping people. This purpose has driven me from the day I left the womb, and from day one, I knew I'd become a doctor. There was really no other profession or livelihood that I envisioned for myself.

Growing up in upstate New York in a small house in Tonawanda, I spent summer nights chasing fireflies and collecting them in jars for my mother, much like any other child, before she would promptly tell me to release the poor things. I was fascinated when a neighbor painted on his arm with the lower abdomen of one, but could never feel comfortable participating in killing them for a temporary moment of wonder. In this respect, I've had reverence for life from a young age.

My Irish-born paternal grandfather died of rheumatic heart disease aged 52 when I was just a toddler, and I suspect that, subconsciously, this imprinted in my brain the instinct to one day become a cardiologist. Another blessing from my childhood involves my paternal aunt's husband, Dr. Al Santos, a cardiologist from Brazil. I fondly remember completing rounds with him at the hospital where he taught students and residents, asking questions and taking in the culture of medicine and healthcare.

I have leaped at any opportunity to positively touch lives through medicine ever since. When my wife finished nursing school we moved for a time to Toronto, Ontario, where her parents lived. During that time, I was finishing medical school and worked on my elective with the Toronto Hospital for Sick Children. I convinced Dr. Robert Salter to let me scrub in on surgeries even though students traditionally were only allowed to observe. At that time, I'd waited two decades for my chance to save lives and I refused to wait another day.

From Precocious to Ferocious

Cardiology called to me for a variety of reasons, not the least of which was the fact that during my first few years practicing medicine, I noticed that at least half of internal medicine was cardiovascular disease. What's more, I loved the continually evolving landscape in cardiology and craved the ability to continue participating on an academic level.

In many ways, I've been relentless since I was a child. I finished top of the class in medical school during my clinical years and 12th out of 199 students during the entire four years. In academic medicine, I was one of the youngest program directors in cardiology and one of the youngest division heads in cardiology when I was the Chief of Cardiology at the University of Missouri in Kansas City. It's fair to say that since I was young, I've been rather precocious.

The drive to excel continued throughout my career, and although I've had exhausting periods of my life - particularly during my first residency in Michigan in a town of two thousand people - I've been compelled to excel in every arena that matters to me. I've run marathons in all fifty states and my wife and I are proud to be within range of the weight we were when we were eighteen; with her beating me out ever so slightly.

Despite the censorship and defamation that I have endured over the past couple of years (which I'll address later in this chapter), I've always been considered a medical doctor with very high standing. I'm the most published person in the world in my field (the interface between kidney and heart disease) in history. I have reached the highest stature of academic medicine and I've lectured before the US FDA, the European Medicine Association Agency, and the New York Academy of Sciences; I've taught and traveled worldwide. In 2007, I was the main presenter at a US Congressional oversight panel for the FDA on a major product label expansion.

I have fifty-six peer-reviewed publications on the pandemic, particularly with regards to the treatment of the infection, and over seven hundred and seventy overall publications in The National Library of Medicine, plus an additional one thousand-plus overall medical communications. I've served on two dozen data safety monitoring boards for large pharmaceutical, device, and in vitro diagnostic studies and I consider myself both an expert on COVID-19 as well as drug, device, and biological agent safety. As proof, just hours before sitting down to write this chapter for my new colleagues at The Wellness Company, I provided testimony to the Texas Senate Committee on Health and Human Services on July 27, 2022, and previously testified in that courtroom on March 10, 2021.

But, my friends, there is no accolade that compares to the transcendental moment I detail at the end of my recent book, *The Courage to Face COVID-19*, co-authored with John Leake. On January 23, 2022, I gave an address at the Lincoln Memorial looking across the reflection pool to the Washington Monument. My enthusiasm for medical scholarship, my compassion for humanity, and my duty to uphold the integrity of our Constitutional Republic all synchronized in that moment; and at that point I'd transformed into a defender of civil liberties.

Today you'll read stories about heroes of mine, some of whom are included in this chapter, and the rest of whom are co-authoring this book with me. Some of these heroes, such as Dr. Richard Amerling, are people I have worked alongside and trusted for decades. Others I've gained as friends and peers during the fight of the past few years. And one thing that nobody can deny; not Dr. Amerling, not my children nor my wife, is that the pandemic drew out qualities in me that I didn't know I had. Alas, I've always excelled in my field and taken care of my body and my family, but I've become crystal clear on my purpose. My ability to convey that purpose as a staunch defender of civil liberties to large groups of individuals has surprised even me.

Thanks to the chaos, I've been honored to deliver hope, understanding, and a new resolve to people. I've learned that we've got to get through this and that we're going to win, but we can only achieve this if we do it together. I've learned what the Kennedy children learned from a young age: that there is no greater honor that they could have than to be alive during a time of great controversy; to play a role in the resolution of crisis. I am truly blessed with the honor of this crisis in history, and I'm part of the resolution. And so are you.

Now Boys, Give 'Em Watts!

As a child, I read the historical accounts of our Founding Fathers with rapt awe for their pioneering and unflinching bravery. In many civil war reenactments, the highlight of the performance is an interpretation of a story about The Reverend Caldwell of the First Presbyterian Church.

Legend has it that The Reverend's wife was shot and killed through a window during the first few days of battle; perhaps whilst nursing their baby, as many versions of the story tell. In response, Reverend

Caldwell joined the Colonial Regiment and found that the colonists were short on wadding to load shot into their muskets. So, the Reverend ran into his church and reemerged carrying stacks of hymnals so that the troops could use the sheets in place of wadding. Because most of the psalms were written by Isaac Watts, Caldwell is now immortalized for his legendary cry encouraging the troops: "Now boys, give 'em Watts!"

The images of brave colonists and soldiers in other crises in history inspired me throughout my childhood. I wondered often if I'd have been one of those brave dissidents who fought for our freedom. I know now that I would "give 'em Watts."

Today, as I lay my head down at night, I sleep well knowing that I have risen to the challenge and I possess an inordinate amount of energy to keep fighting. I hope that by the end of this book, you'll too join me in the peace that comes from fighting for good.

I Think We Should Take These Statements Seriously

From the very beginning of the pandemic, I felt that this chaotic time had clear spiritual aspects to it. Often people ask me if I believe there's an Illuminati or a great conspiracy. In fact, in the most downloaded show in the history of his podcast (there I go being precocious again), Joe Rogan even asked me if I believe that there's "a conspiracy." Others quietly ask me if there's a plan for global genocide. I sense they don't want to know the answer either way; there's undoubtedly a morbid fascination in our culture to know the evil agendas and perverted habits of dark forces that lurk in the shadows.

Nevertheless, I privately chuckle at the naivete of the question. How does one presume that I've intercepted the memoirs and been privy to the secret chamber meetings of the global elite?

Wait a second, I have. In fact, so have you.

My co-author in *Courage to Face COVID-19,* John Leake, aptly writes that we should take all public utterances very seriously. I couldn't agree with him more.

- When Bill Gates and the Gates Foundation stated in a TED Talk (aired over a decade ago now) that a method to reduce the world's population is mass vaccination, I think we should take that statement seriously.

- When Gates says that the next decade is the decade of the vaccine, bragging on camera about vaccination being a great investment with a "twenty to one return;" I think we should take that statement seriously.

- When the Coalition of Epidemic Preparedness Innovations, or CEPI, was formed by the Gates Foundation and the World Economic Forum in 2017, they published a business plan stating that there would be pandemics and that as each one comes along, their business plan would be the development of vaccines. I think we should take that seriously.

- When Executive Chairman of the World Economic Forum Klaus Schwab published *The Great Reset* in 2020 just a few months after the onset of the crisis, saying in it that this is an opportunity to reset a new world order through a context of a health emergency, I think we should take these statements seriously.

- When Vineet Menachery as first author and senior author Ralph Baric published in *PNAS* "SARS-like WIV1-CoV poised for human emergence" and in *Nature Medicine*, "A SARS-like cluster of circulating bat coronaviruses shows potential for human emergence," the publication of these statements in credible scientific journals means that we should take this seriously.

- On October 19, 2019, the Johns Hopkins Center for Public Security collaborated with the Bill and Melinda Gates Foundation and the World Economic Forum on a Pandemic Simulation Exercise. I think we should take that seriously. Folks, it's a scientific reality that they knew what was going on.

There is widespread corruption that has occurred, and is still occurring, at the level of international organizations such as the World Economic Forum, the World Health Organization, GAVI, SEPI, the Coalition for Epidemic Preparedness and Innovation, the Eco-Health Alliance, The National Institutes of Health, the CDC, the US FDA, the Wellcome Trust and Gates Foundations, the Rockefeller Foundation, the CCP; there appears to be a syndicate if you will.

The final arenas for fairness are through our judicial and legal systems. The Biopharmaceutical Complex has swept through institution after institution; through the major medical colleges, through hospitals, through the health system, through large corporations, and now it's in the courts.

No matter what you call it, this appears to be a wide-scale battle of Good vs. Evil. During the Revolutionary War, we understand that approximately 3 percent of the population fought, 10 percent of the population supported those who fought, and the rest of society stood back and watched. You may wonder why people don't "wake up." You may have even wished that a few quadruple-masked "Karens" would just take their fourth booster already and leave you alone indefinitely. You may be biting your nails at the thought of your employer requiring masks again soon. And all this, naturally, would drive an awakened person crazy.

But understand that in every single historical battle of Good vs. Evil, there is a relatively small number of people on the side of Good… and a disproportionately large number of people on the side of Evil. Our numbers may be small, but you're not alone. What's more, together we don't have to evangelize, convert, or even engage with 85 percent of the unawakened population to win this war. We are powerful, together.

The Biopharmaceutical Complex

Imagine for a moment that there's an invading army marching down your street. Your neighbors are safely tucked away in their houses, peering through half-closed windows. Inevitably, there are a small number of people that jump out in the street and try to fight the army. There are also a large number of people who close the blinds, lock the doors, and try to weather out the storm in invisible silence—the majority most likely. Some people would call out to the people in the street, warning their defenders, "Get inside! Don't make waves! Don't try to fight them!" Those are the ones that can really get under our skin.

Over the past two years, several people have said to me, "Why don't you stop? Why can't you be quiet and let this happen? You can't control this. It's too big."

During those moments, I remember my colonial countrymen. Like them, we are faced with an invading army; an army which I call the Biopharmaceutical Complex. Fundamentally, it's categorized and manifested by incompetence at the highest levels of our medical institutions. It's the phenomenon of healthy economics being perverted in medicine.

Healthy economic forces revolve around competition. This is what allows us to secure the best product at the best price. In medicine, that involves extensive research and development, testing, and multiple carriers of a product, treatment, or medicine. It makes you safer and it saves lives. Among other things, we have witnessed the decline of healthy economic forces over the past two years. We are watching as Pfizer and Moderna dominate their market with no effective competition.

We've watched as tens of millions of doses of the COVID-19 "vaccine," were wasted as a result of pre-purchasing. We've seen the growth of Remdesivir, an intravenous polymerase inhibitor that didn't just fail to reduce mortality during the Ebola trials but caused kidney and liver injury.

And yet, it's being prescribed in hospitals to unsuccessfully treat COVID-19 even as I write this paragraph. The European Society of Critical Care advised against the use of Remdesivir. The World Health Authority recommends that it is not used. And yet, here in America, hospitals were given a 20 percent bonus on the hospital payments when they used it; like a tip on the bill.

Hospital administrators, it appears, could not resist the financial incentives that the US passed down, and perhaps 2.5 million Americans were "treated" with this failed drug. Analysis suggests we lost a million American lives, and much of that was contributed through what we call a perverse incentive. The Biopharmaceutical Complex has a stranglehold on our entire system. And so, The Wellness Company is spearheading a new one.

A Call for Courage

There has never been a checkbox on an application that I have ever filled out that measured courage. Not one. And after my considerably successful career, that surprises me more than any other thing my mentors and teachers failed to impart to me in medical school. We think of soldiers, firemen, and police officers as needing courage to fight fires, detain bad guys and even fight our enemies. But as a doctor, there is no checkbox or terms and conditions that prioritize courage. Alas, in the medical profession there are many heroes, but courage is optional.

I'm sad to say that it's really, very rare. Part of my personal mission with The Wellness Company is to enlist more courageous medical professionals in the fight.

As of today, we're not fighting a battle where bullets are flying. Rather, it's a war of information. People are being injured and even sacrificed at the end of a hypodermic needle. They're being injured because they are denied therapy and die unnecessarily horrific deaths on the mechanical ventilator. It's not bullets being physically fired at one another, but more people have died from the COVID-19 jab than died in the Vietnam War. Make no mistake about it, this is, indeed, a war.

On that note, over the past two years, I've been tempted to overthink and even become bitter at the lack of medical professionals who have adopted the position of compassionate care; trying to help people through illness and avoid hospitalization and death. Without any reservations, I know that I took the correct position; that there was no other correct position. It's now clear that the investigative COVID-19 shots are causing vast numbers of injuries, disabilities, and deaths. The new mission is to engage those you love and urge them to stop taking them.

The estimate is that approximately eighty-two percent of Americans have already succumbed to taking one of the shots. Worldwide, that number is closer to two-thirds; two-thirds of the world allows an injection into their bodies without questioning the contents; without any assurances on long-term safety. Rather than courageously speaking up for themselves or taking personal responsibility to safeguard their very lives, they surrendered.

There is only one explanation. It's Good vs. Evil. There is no ambiguity.

The Superbowl of Internal Medicine

Countless medical professionals chose to ignore their own discernment and take the investigative COVID-19 shot because of pressure in their institutions. Others are awakened and yet choose not to speak out. A friend recently recalled a private conversation she had with her son's pediatrician, during which the pediatrician stated: "If you want me to recommend against the pediatric COVID-19, I simply can't. The American Pediatric Association recommends it. The CDC recommends it. And you know what? I have a family to feed. My hands are tied."

This is not courage. It's homicide. In May 2021, I told Tucker Carlson in an interview that, starting in 2020, we had the opportunity to witness the Superbowl of Internal Medicine at the onset of the Sars Cov 2 outbreak.

I'm on the field. A few doctors have joined me. A few stood on the sidelines. Many more didn't even bother to play the game or even heckled from the opposing team's side. Some headed for the exits. Sars Cov 2 and COVID-19 were the great separators of heroes from villains; of the courageous from the cowardly.

I distinctly remember telling a colleague that when I walk through a hallway at my major medical center every day, these doctors look down at the ground when I pass. I'm still there just about every day. Those physicians, many of whom are my former friends, cannot lift their heads or look me in the eye. They're ashamed of themselves. They ran for the exits. They heckled from the opposing team's side. In some cases, they know they have done something wrong, but it seems like they cannot identify precisely what that is or was. Indeed, they are in some form of trance, some sort of mass psychosis.

I imagine that this is similar to a doctor who participated in ushering both Jews and non-Jews to the gas chambers. I once heard a story of a church in Germany that would play the organ louder when the trains passed carrying prisoners to the concentration camps, drowning out the misery. Similarly, people have anesthetized their own convictions, common sense, or intellectual curiosities with Netflix, booze, or never-ending rabbit holes in the dark corners of the internet, fascinating over conspiracy theories that can albeit be fascinating but not productive.

Doctors are not immune to such frivolities or anesthetization. The doctors who have participated in ill-advised treatments have been in a daze–a trance. These doctors refused to answer calls for patients with COVID-19. They refused to provide early or effective treatments. They refused to prescribe safe drugs like ivermectin or hydroxychloroquine, leaving it up to courageous small retail pharmacies or telemedicine groups like what we're building here with The Wellness Company.

These doctors went against the advice of the World Health Organization, published in November of 2020, warning that Remdesivir was more likely to result in kidney injury, liver damage, or even death. And yet, these doctors administered that death sentence because it was "on a protocol" that came down through the US Department of Health and Human Services, pocketing their twenty percent bonus on the hospital bill. In some ways, they sold their souls, and their treachery will be examined in schools of public health for decades to come.

The Second Hero

Like many of my peers in this book, I have taken precious little time off since the onset of the pandemic. I was working on an investigation on drug applications and received a sizable research grant organized by my research team to fight the pandemic. I've published critical papers on early treatment and was involved in the White House on Emergency Use Authorization Extension attempts, and I was the overall principal investigator on grants that were put forward for Ramatroban as well as in support of the Immodulon vaccine programs. Scientifically, my craving for professional challenge and innovation has been sated.

I answer calls from people who need help, and I still make house calls. I respond to people who need help because that's what I do. It's the work I've desired to do since birth. I'm involved in a communication system that is in its third year of operation with approximately two hundred other doctors who are sharing scientific advancements. I'm also highly active on social media; at least where I haven't been censored. I'm an active member of many grassroots organizations. I model bravery by letting Americans see my mug nearly every night on the news. I am bold, relentless, and I'm not going to stop until this crisis is closed.

And still, there's another hero on whose shoulders I stand, and that's Senator Ron Johnson. In my book, *Courage to Face COVID-19,* I share the following words in the acknowledgments: "Finally, I would like to give a very special thanks to Senator Ron Johnson (R-WI). In my view, he is the finest US Senator in history for his courageous stand on behalf of suffering patients and compassionate doctors who fought against all odds during this crisis."

Johnson is a defender of the doctors who have chosen to play in this arena. I've been in his chambers and testified twice under his direction. He sees things clearly, respects the clinical decision-making of doctors, and is unafraid to call out corruption and the co-opting of the US Senate and House of Representatives with regard to the Biopharmaceutical Complex. Senator Johnson is a real American patriot.

In the spirit of Senator Johnson, I've fought another private battle over the past two years, and it's largely more political than anything I thought I'd personally encounter.

Namely, there is a rumor circulating that I have been discredited, which I am here to extinguish. I have, in truth, never been discredited or challenged by any person of any medical standing in the world. All the forms of censorship I have encountered come through anonymous, uncredentialed internet identities, probably consisting of robotic programs; not people of recognizable standing.

Interestingly, the fact-checkers on the internet and social media can be traced back to the Poynter Institute; put on your tinfoil hats again because the Poynter Institute is linked to none other than the Gates Foundation. Anonymous people within the Gates Foundation are, in all probability, my biggest opponents.

I've never received an email from a doctor with any standard in medicine. Most attacks on me have been via email, certified letter, or email. I've been stripped of two editorships of peer-reviewed journals without phone calls or meetings. I was stripped of two professorships in universities in my metro area with no due process, no faculty senate, and no review of a different point of view. Not even a courtesy phone call.

These are remarkable historical events and today we'll use them to note that in a free and civil society, we should be up in arms that events like these take place. One of your responsibilities after reading this book is to relish what free speech you have and to never, ever stop fighting for the honor of having it.

The Fight Against Free Speech

In another more political sense, I've been deployed as a soldier in the fight for Good vs. Evil for my own job security. I'm an active practitioner, always available to my clients, 24/7. I've been in internal medicine and cardiology practice continuously now since starting in 1991. I have a perfect track record with state licensure and with the American Board of Internal Medicine, which I electively recertify every ten years, effectively putting my professional status on the line with recertification exams.

On May 26, 2022, I received a letter from the American Board of Internal Medicine stating I was to undergo a review for potential disciplinary sanction. They pointed out that they had reviewed public statements I'd made as the lead witness in the US Senate on Pandemic Response on two occasions. I've been a testifying expert in multiple state senate hearings. I'm a frequent contributor on many major media outlets; including Fox News, Newsmax, Victory Channel, and One America Voice on ABC. I also have my own podcast, *The McCullough Report* on the America Out Loud Platform. I've made innumerable public comments that can be reviewed.

In their letter, the American Board of Internal Medicine wrote, "ABIM has learned that you have made numerous widely reported and disseminated public statements about the purported dangers of or lack of justification for COVID-19 vaccines."

As a doctor, I make many statements regarding many vaccines. I make statements regarding many in vitro diagnostic tests. I make statements regarding therapies. I've obviously made many statements regarding heart and kidney disease.

As I mentioned above, I have over seven hundred and fifty peer-reviewed publications in the National Library of Medicine. Doctors are professionals of public importance, and they have a right to give their analysis and opinion in a public venue on topics of public health importance. That's exactly what I've done. However, the American Board of Internal Medicine, in their review, has selected five statements that I made under oath in the Texas Senate on March 10, 2021. As an expert testifying under oath - as I've done many times - I can tell you that that activity is taken with the utmost sincerity. It's sworn under oath; the whole truth, nothing but the truth, and that questions are answered to the best of the ability of the witness.

This action taken by the American Board of Internal Medicine is unprecedented. It is unprecedented that a professional giving their opinion under oath would be subject to reprisal from a physician organization regarding the statements made. That means that, in this current era, a nurse, a respiratory therapist, an engineer, a lawyer, a patient, or anyone who makes a statement under oath is potentially in the crosshairs for professional or personal reprisal or damage. I think everyone should be alarmed by this development.

Censorship is a direct threat to our constitutional rights. It's working to unite people across a broad spectrum of party lines by dividing them. A worldwide threat, it's wielded by many different parties in many different countries, whether they're democracies, theocracies, or communistic countries. New Zealand Prime Minister Jacinda Ardern said in July 2022, "We will continue to be your single source of truth."

This is highly reminiscent of Nazi Germany and the office of propaganda, where the regime indicated that it would be the single source of truth. This is dangerously close to the single TV station available in communist North Korea. And yet, these countries are held out as civil democracies. Everyone should be disturbed by this.

Censorship also unites people across party lines, as we've seen with the ultra-right-wing Steve Bannon and liberal CNN commentator Naomi Wolf. Seeing them work together excites and inspires me, not because of their political philosophies, but because of their willingness to step across the aisle for the greater good. Oddly, censorship unites others in a way that restores my appreciation for humanity; and I am already a big fan of humans (just not the nefarious and complicit ones I've named in this chapter). For instance, precisely because I have detractors, my supporters are closer to my message and closer to one another. Indeed, there is a sea of ten thousand supporters for each living detractor. As for the online detractors, that's a more incalculable number.

Now visualize with me a world that adopts a fair, balanced, and critical review of the COVID-19 global vaccination program. Imagine a medical community committed above all else to the patient's best interest. Imagine that the pediatrician I mentioned earlier had said, "there's no discernable benefit of COVID-19 vaccination for children, and so I refuse to recommend this injection."

The Court Coup

As I've illustrated, a sizable percentage of Americans understand that the COVID-19 investigative gene-based treatment which has been labeled as a "vaccine" does not work. At least 18 percent of Americans rejected even one shot. Reports suggest that only 5 percent of parents chose to inoculate their small children under five years of age.

These empirical facts have given many people the permission needed to wake up. And yet, an even greater percentage of people are digging in their heels, refusing to see this evidence that the COVID-19 injection simply does not work as intended, if at all. Later, my colleague here at The Wellness Company, Dr. Harvey Risch, will fascinate you in his discussion of Negative Efficacy.

I wasn't merely fascinated with biological sciences since birth, but also with the human condition. I'm appalled at how many people seem to justify the suffering of others through the risk of the injection simply because they have; subconsciously they seem to feel entitled to impose medical tyranny on others because they've taken the risk and, somehow, they seem to think that others should, too. That's a fight in our courts that requires your support. If you aren't fighting in the courts, find somebody who is and donate to them. They need you. We need you.

As for me, I have the honor of fighting back by assisting on over one hundred cases of various litigation from major issues on President

Biden's nationwide vaccine mandates. In fact, my testimony was relied upon by Judge Doughty in the federal courts, which propelled that case to the Supreme Court of the United States. Because of my testimony, four out of the five Biden mandates were overturned.

As I sit here in my study writing, I'm reminded that just yesterday, in late July 2022, we learned that an International Guardsman in Kansas won in the courts to uphold his preference for religious exemption. That case relied on my testimony. As a plaintiff or defendant, I'm actively involved in about a dozen cases.

One famously is against Twitter. I, alongside my fellow plaintiffs Dr. Robert Malone and Dr. Bryan Tyson, learned through a release of documents from a related activity that the CDC was actively meeting with Twitter and developing plans for censorship and standard operating procedures for the reprisal of those holding Twitter accounts. Simply put, if accounts or account holders were not in line with the government's false narrative on COVID-19 and pandemic response, there would be censorship or reprisal. Consider how extraordinary these observations are: a US Government entity took part in a conspiracy operating against citizens of the US and citizens of the world.

The Court of Public Opinion

We have addressed a coup in the courts in favor of Big Pharma, Big Tech, Big Government, and Big Finance, also identified by the heroic Russiagate whistleblower Retired Colonel John Mills as the "Four Corners of Deceit" in his book *The Nation Will Follow*. One court that seems to be open is the court of public opinion.

Here is some more good news. It is clear that if the public declines any more of the COVID-19 jabs then the entire program fails. The entire shroud of a false narrative, this entire operation of censorship and reprisal; it all falls. The court of public opinion will work in our favor.

With the COVID-19 investigative gene-based treatments, errantly called vaccines, resulting in large numbers of deaths, heart damage, blood clots, neurological damage, and hematologic damage, there has ignited a global call for these products to be taken off the market.

On June 11, 2022, the World Council for Health Pharmacovigilance Report called for the removal of all vaccines for COVID-19 from the market. Read that back, because you won't hear about it on the news (for that matter, you probably shouldn't be watching the mainstream news without a diligent filter, anyway). This is not a subtle message to the vaccine stakeholders nor the entire Biopharmaceutical Complex; they are on the receiving end of a very clear message from doctors in positions of authority and from patients and concerned citizens who have either been damaged by these vaccines or who are fearful of future damage.

When the world rejects vaccinations, the program will fail.

When the COVID-19 investigative "vaccines" are taken off the market, there will be a worldwide holiday. My heart swells in my chest at the thought of seeing joy and relief in my colleagues' faces when the menace finally ends and the remaining shots are destroyed. At that moment, and I do believe we will see that moment, we will be more united than ever.

In this book, my colleagues will continue to illustrate how your heroes and mine are leveraging free speech amidst unprecedented censorship to awaken that small but critical mass of doctors and laypeople. Just moments ago, I learned of a woman who respectfully asked a Hollywood director if he'd considered petitioning his union to protect his medical freedom. He said, "Friend, I can't tell you how many people in Hollywood showed up to the Oscars with forged vaccine cards. But people are scared to admit that they've resorted to fraud in order to protect their medical freedom." The conversation evolved into a meaningful and philosophical discussion about why so many directors, actors, and agents haven't had the courage to hold the line, refuse to relinquish their medical freedom, and petition their unions to honor that freedom.

Today, that respected Hollywood director is encouraged to act with integrity, honor, and bravery in the face of tyranny. What will come of this? What if we all engaged our fellow Americans to relish instead of relinquishing what free speech we have left before it's forbidden to even ask these questions; before we're afraid of the CDC knocking on our doors with needles… or muzzles… in hand?

I perform all my work pro bono in the courts, even if a case goes all the way to the Supreme Court. But perhaps you don't have to go that far. Perhaps your presence at school board meetings will intimidate and derail bad actors just enough to protect your children until our critical mass overturns rampant public school abuses.

What will you do today to politely and elegantly engage your friends, families, audiences, and peers? What fight are you ready to take up with those school boards? Within your county's family court? On your election boards? How are you being a good steward of your audiences on social media, even if it's "merely" a few hundred LinkedIn connections?

Remember, tomorrow could be too late.

The Third Hero

This chapter will close with a spotlight on our third hero. That hero is you.

Let's take a moment to explore how we'll engage our families and children right now to be victorious in today's fight as well as in future generations. Let's analyze the villains that hold us back and stifle our march to progress, as the awareness of them gives us the ability to overcome them.

I'll remind you that in winter war years, such as during the Second World War, we enjoy generations of spring and summer. As a literate adult in today's war on information and medical freedom, you're officially enlisted and deployed. Provided we are good stewards of the critical mass we're building, we will leave a legacy for our grandchildren just as our heroic grandparents did for us.

Villain #1: Shame

My own family has been burned by the COVID-19 injection. In particular, two elderly family members couldn't come to the US from Canada without the injections. I'm not preaching from a podium; I'm here lamenting alongside you. Although my nuclear family was blessed to be able to avoid the shots, people I love did, in fact, cave.

It is with immense sadness that I tell you that one of those pressured members of my family has already died. We cannot know if it was directly because of the shot due to his advanced age, but what I do assure you of is this: he didn't want that shot. Still fresh in my mind, I regularly place my feet on the floor in the morning and see his face in my mind's eye. I'm fighting for him.

There is one fate slightly better than death, according to Dr. David Hawkins' *Map of Consciousness*, and that's shame. He refers to shame as "perilously proximate to death" and "conscious suicide" in his posthumously published 2020 book, *The Map of Consciousness Explained.*

On the subject of shame, a younger person in my family took two shots in January 2021 and then simply refused to talk about it. We are not a family of timid voices; this indicated to me that there must have been a degree of shame around the actions of that family member. That same family member also knew that I'm not an "anti-vaxxer;" - I've taken them all myself - but it shows you that there's something different about this shot; it begets a low vibration of consciousness. It compels the shot taker to furnish excuses such as "I was trying to protect other people," which is a phrase that in a cowardly way negates personal responsibility.

In the summer of 2021, the CDC publicly stated that the COVID-19 injection does not protect other people, acknowledging that these investigative gene-based therapies do not prevent the spread of infection. The CDC, most likely reticent, revealed to us that based on empirical data, the "vaccines" do not halt the spread of COVID-19, and taking them does not protect anybody else. Now, that same younger person in my family took a booster but waited a full eighteen months. In his case, he felt it was essential to navigate the next steps in his career.

Hearing that, I'm further incited. That second administration of a booster shot was now made with my family member's knowledge of eighteen months of data showing heart damage, blood clots, FDA warnings slapped on the drugs, and death. The consent form indicates clearly that side effects can range from a sore arm to death.

This is what I refer to as a game of Russian Roulette. With all the evidence we have before us, if you're taking a COVID-19 shot or booster you are literally saying, "I'm either gonna regret this, potentially with my life, or I'm gonna get lucky." Personally, I've never been a gambler.

In just one case, a person in my family willingly took the shot. This athlete is in his mid-50s and, although having had four shots, he contracted COVID-19 while traveling to Europe. Everything was taken away from him and he was put into a COVID-19 hotel in Germany. He was allowed to progressively sicken and became seriously ill. By God's grace, he avoided a mechanical ventilator and survived, most likely thanks to his exceptional physical shape. Four shots. Zero protection. Hospitalized and receiving no early treatment whatsoever.

Now, what shall we take away from this personal story about my own family? Well, for starters, evidence suggests to me that like my three injected family members, if people had a choice, the COVID-19 injection would not be taken at all. Many of my family members have received the McCullough Protocol and have received early treatment in something I call the sequenced multi-drug therapy. Every one of them experienced the prompt resolution of symptoms, including the elderly—one of whom contracted COVID-19 in an independent living facility and recovered in five days. Note that the quadruple-vaxxed mid-50s triathlete ended up in the hospital with COVID-19 and no early treatment. I trust you can interpret this in a way that elevates your life and your family's.

The Wellness Company is here to help you locate the protocol that you feel is best to fight COVID-19 when you visit us at www.twc.health.

Villain #2: Entitlement

There is no greater way to elevate our Third Hero than with a call to self-reliance. I'm in a unique position to discuss self-reliance. I'm in what's referred to as the Sandwich Generation. I never took a penny from my parents, earning income from the age of 12 as a paperboy with my brother and paying my way through medical school with a combination of grants, hard work, and a decent salary upon leaving school that helped me resolve loans fairly quickly.

And yet, although I haven't relied on my parents, I'm responsible for their well-being. In addition, my children are part of an entirely different generation, one that often does not earn their way through a McDonald's drive-thru, let alone college. And so, folks in the Sandwich Generation are responsible for both their parents and their kids. This is a unique position that has given me a gift of perspective that I will offer you today.

Since the age of 12, every dollar I've spent is a dollar I've earned; in New York as a paperboy who delivered papers on foot weekdays and collected money for them on the weekends. When my family moved to Texas whilst I was in high school, I continued as a paperboy but, of course, everything is bigger in Texas. Now I delivered papers on a bike and instead of bringing them to the door, I developed a competitive arm throwing them up the driveways of much bigger homes and yards. I'd treat myself periodically to a burger or a milkshake and think, *well, that's pretty great*. It just tasted better when I earned it myself.

Shame is a fascinating and tragic part of most humans' existence. Another tragedy is an entitlement, subconsciously or otherwise. You see, a large number of people in their mid-20s today haven't earned a single dollar they spend. They can't even remember their phone passwords, let alone the individual and real-time past due newspaper tabs among one hundred different houses. Where's the pride? Does the kill taste as sweet when you haven't participated in the hunt? As for me, I'll likely never know.

This entire phenomenon of self-reliance represents a cataclysmic shift in family economics that hinges on the concept of personal responsibility. Poetically, personal responsibility is a core foundation of The Wellness Company, if not *the* core foundation. Unlike animals such as horses, humans are biologically reliant on their parents for a number of years after birth. However, that child-rearing phase of life has extended beyond anything we can recall in human history.

Why is this and how does it apply to you? Well for one, allow your kids to enjoy the fruits of a hard day's labor. Have them bake cookies or make lemonade to earn that new drone they've been eyeing. And secondly, consider nurturing your child in the dying art of taking time off. Truly.

The age of information technology, as well as changes in education, have robbed children of their former playtime, imagination-wielding, and "run home before the street lights go on" freedom. In the "paper and pen" decades, we were done with work when we left the office. Most of you reading this book recall the transition from paper and pen to computers. Certainly, at 59 years old, I do.

It's not just adults who are overworked, but kids, too. Education became enormously complex in this age of information. Among other things, children spend more time preparing for college exams than they spend earning money for college. Why is that?

There has been an expansion of willingness to pay. For example, college education used to be paid for either by the student or in a work-study program with which the student would be engaged. In other less frequent situations, students would receive scholarships or loans. In recent decades, college education became one of the most inflated cost items in the American and Canadian budgets, the root cause of which is taxpayer-backed and subsidized student loans. The cost of a college education far exceeds the cost of transportation, mining for oil and gas in the extractive industries sector, financial services, food, and more. Once college costs grew beyond the reach of work-study and the concept of "paying my way through college" died before the grunge era was complete, there was no longer a game worth winning. If there's no way to pay for college through hard work, why put in all that hard work?

What would "Deep Thoughts" by Dr. McCullough be without a note about the larger and more nefarious economic forces at play in this scenario? During the 80s, 90s, and past 2000, parents had college savings accounts. However, the cost of college education mysteriously began to increase in proportion to the money that was squirreled away in these accounts. In essence, tuition was going to drain these accounts dry. And that's what's happened.

This confluence of factors has led to the fact that there is virtually no child in America who can claim that every dollar they've spent was self-earned from 12, as I and so many others like me did.

As for the average young person - certainly in middle and upper-class America - every dollar they have ever spent has been earned by their parents. And so, therefore, one couldn't expect a young person now to possess a high degree of self-reliance; and it isn't entirely their fault. Nevertheless, what happens to a society when people have become dependent versus self-reliant?

That question has already been answered: the complete hijacking of our medical system by the Biopharmaceutical Complex. And the next question is this: how do we fight those bandits? My colleagues and I are answering that question, starting with this very book. We are aligning to answer every need you have, at least in outpatient care, supplementation, and education. We are building and aligning ourselves with providers of the legal resources (now that I'm apparently an expert plaintiff and defendant) so that you can protect everything from your right to breathe clean air to your job… and most especially, so that you will be empowered and prepared to protect your children from the fate too many innocent children suffered this year. Because I am a father, a brother, a husband, and a son sandwiched between the needs and care of so many generations, I know your struggles. I'm with you.

Villain #3: Remorse

The question that makes me chuckle, "do you think there's a worldwide conspiracy?" is dangerously close to the question "will two thirds of the population die from the shot?" This question doesn't make me chuckle. It makes my heart heavy.

The truth is this: I don't know what's going to happen, but we must be prepared for death. Our CDC is telling us that over thirteen thousand Americans have died after taking the shot, and we know, if COVID-19 death reporting is anything to go by, that could be subject to a vast underreporting.

One paper by Pentas Atos and Seligman from Columbia indicates that the upper bound confidence interval, that is the higher side of a likely or probable range of people who have died after the shot, could be as high as one hundred and eighty-seven thousand souls. Lincoln National has reported 63 percent excess mortality, and they know it's from something other than COVID-19. To put this in perspective, an extraordinary one-in-two-hundred-year event would beget a 10 percent increase in mortality. I know of no other time in recorded history where mortality has been this high.

I don't see how these sobering figures can be suppressed. On one level, maybe people actually do know what they're getting themselves into. Maybe they say, "Well, so-and-so took a risk and a gamble. He knew the parachute was not gonna open for everybody." Others suspect that the deaths are suppressed.

And yet I see a third phenomenon: the sudden emergence of remorse. Take Ernesto Ramirez, a father in South Texas whose child died due to myocarditis. Ernesto immediately recognized the mistake and publicly came out, imploring other parents to take heed on the back of his tragic loss. Ernesto came out of the trance. He's awake. He knows something bad is going on. And so do you.

Another interesting case study is that of Dr. Robert Malone. Malone holds patents in the development of the messenger RNA of lipid particle technology. Theoretically, he could have been in line for a Nobel Prize if these shots would have saved the world. Although he and his wife already had the illness, they took the shot. When he had side effects, he realized that these are dangerous products. Just like Ramirez, Dr. Malone emerged from the trance. He publicly expressed his regret and remorse.

There's a lot to learn from these courageous examples about how we must carry on. If you're reading this and you have taken one or more shots, I pray that, like Malone and Ramirez, you have now awoken from the trance and are ready to speak up about the dangers we can now scientifically indicate.

As brave warriors in the fight to take back our medical freedom and overcome the Biopharmaceutical Complex, let us take note of Ramirez and Malone. Let us mimic their courage, vaccinated or not, and devote our hearts and actions to the duty of speaking up and speaking out. You may save a life or two.

We will devote the final thoughts in this chapter to a refreshing topic: that of my personal intentions for you and your family's wellness, and the strategies needed to fight back for the benefit of you and your family.

Strategy #1: Become Your Own Medical Advocate

I want each and every one of you reading this book to schedule an appointment with your doctor. Go over your medication, your history, your supplements, and your goals. Now ask your doctor one question: "Should I take these COVID-19 investigative gene based therapies?"

Allow your doctor to answer before you enter into any debate or argument over data. If your doctor says yes, your response should be, "I don't feel as if these "vaccines" are safe enough for me." Doctors need to hear the sentiment that patients do not feel that these are safe enough. They need to receive that feedback over and over again.

Once you allow your doctor to answer, simply restate your position. "I'm sorry, Doctor. These may be safe enough for you, but they're not safe enough for me or my family." And then, just leave it there. Don't walk out in a huff; patients still need their doctors. Don't refuse to set foot in a hospital ever again and find a shaman who's going to heal your chronic disease with vomit-inducing teas. As a cardiologist and internal medicine doctor, I sometimes prescribe pharmaceuticals. My patients express concern over medications all the time. I don't abandon them. They don't leave me. We engage in an open and honest consultative process that puts the best interests of the patient at the forefront.

In the world we're creating, my colleagues and I in this book are providing brand new alternatives for many aspects of medicine. However, patients who are deep into various diseases will need their own personal physician team.

You must express your feelings that the shot is not safe enough for you, just like you would with a medicine that you're not comfortable with.

A reasonable doctor would not force medicine on a patient that they are not comfortable with. The same goes for these investigative gene products that are called "vaccines." But you as the patient must articulate your position. Your health is your wealth.

In this manner, you must become self-reliant. And for some, that's going to require a bit of bravery, too.

Strategy #2: Avoid Alcohol and Excess Weight

Over twenty years ago, I made the empowered decision to quit drinking alcohol. I note that it was empowered because I didn't have a gun to my head, so to speak. What I did have was the clarity of mind to assess the risks versus benefits, coming eventually to the resolve to quit.

Alcohol is linked to the later development of dementia, macular degeneration, oral and esophageal cancers, liver disease, traumatic accidents, and a common cardiovascular problem called atrial fibrillation. Research indicates that it may be the most important determinant of heart failure. What's more, alcohol is the single leading cause of a bad night's sleep; it disrupts sleep architecture.

The 28-Day Alcohol-Free Challenge by Andy Ramage and Ruari Fairbairns is the story of two men who lived in England and drank more than their fair share. In their book, they chronicle the benefits of ending a drinking habit over twenty-eight days. In short, they slept better, lost weight, experienced a boost in their energy, and a reduction in symptoms of anxiety. While I'm not making such broad, sweeping medical claims as those, here's what we know based on the science.

It does take about twenty-eight days to restore normal sleep architecture after the ill effects of alcohol. It also takes approximately that long to lose the weight we gain from alcohol consumption. You see, alcohol leads to weight gain because it provides calories that cannot be used as energy. Therefore, every calorie present in a milliliter of alcohol gets deposited into fat and is, along with fructose, a major cause of fatty liver disease. Similarly to quitting smoking, dropping alcohol has a myriad of benefits that outweigh the surmountable task of adjusting your social habits, or perhaps even your friends. Losing weight is gratifying in and of itself and can be life-altering. Shockingly, only approximately 10 percent of people in adulthood are within their high school weight.

Over time, maintaining a weight comparable to our weight at the age of 18 (in the case of a healthy 18-year-old) results in a ninety percent reduction in the risk for diabetes, high blood pressure, and cardiovascular disease. One will also enjoy the vastly reduced risk of gallbladder disease, kidney stones, and chronic degenerative joint disease.

The vast majority of hip and knee replacements performed worldwide are performed for individuals who live sedentary lifestyles; our joints are simply not designed to manage two hundred pounds or more of weight; they are optimized for weight more along the lines of ninety to a hundred and twenty pounds. Excess weight and a lack of physical conditioning facilitate degenerative joint and lower back disease.

You'll sometimes hear people say, "You can't take your money with you when you die." Clearly, that's true. But another thing I've noticed is that over the decades, the single most important thing to aging people is the musculoskeletal function of their bodies and freedom from pain. As people age, they are much more concerned about chronic knee, hip, or back pain and the misery that causes. I haven't heard any regrets about time spent in the office or money. Rather, the remorse I see in people is far and away a result of not taking sufficient care of their bodies.

Take control, and grow old comfortably.

Strategy #3: Control Your Pain

Allow me to provide you with a short answer to the question you all have: "Dr. McCullough, what can I do if I've already been jabbed?" I hear this all the time.

While The Wellness Company will provide you with many terrific resources, my desperate plea is that you take care of your mind and body in a preventative way going forward.

Let's discuss the symbiotic relationship between the mind and body. The connection is not ephemeral or esoteric; it's very real. I'll use the example of pain.

Pain can be divided into three categories. A third of pain is mechanical pain, like a knife sticking in a wound or bone spurs sticking into muscles and tendons.

Another third is what's called allodynia. With allodynia, one experiences normal physical perceptions or nervous signals that go to the brain, but the brain's volume is amplified. In this case, small nuisances in the body feel much more painful than they actually are.

The final third of pain ties everything together. This pain is directly related to the misdirected emotions of anxiety, distress, despair, remorse, loneliness, depression, and chronic fatigue. Regularly, I'm asked about my thoughts on epigenetics or the science of belief. What I know is this: surgeries for painful conditions aren't often helpful unless somebody is suffering from true mechanical pain. In my experience, there is clearly a mind-body connection. A strong body follows a strong mind.

In order to keep my mind and body healthy, I'm diligent in regularly assessing the relationships around me. There is ample published data about happiness, and laughter is a powerful force for positive health. Above all, there is no doubt that connection with and contribution to others is paramount to your healthiest, happiest life. I am blessed to say that the people around me infuse me with so much positive energy and excitement for life that there is rarely a moment I don't have the energy to look darkness in the face and say "bring it on." I'm tireless, but I'm fueled in great part by the quality of the relationships in my life.

Social media offers a touching example of how people unite to bring greater connection with and contribution to others in their lives. Recently, I heard the story of a woman who connected on Telegram with a group of like-minded friends in her otherwise unsupportive and isolating small town. Not only did she find a doctor who ushered her through her own COVID-19 prevention routine, but that same doctor was able to prescribe her grandparents ivermectin "just in case." One of her grandparents was already in assisted living with several chronic problems.

At the advice of a piece of uncensored online information on that Telegram group, her grandparents had also been diligently supplementing with essential vitamins, such as Vitamin D, which the woman mindfully sourced for her grandparents through the advice of a caring naturopath to ensure she wasn't sending the nutritional equivalent of sawdust to her grandparents. When her grandparents fell ill with COVID-19, the woman booked a flight to visit them, assuming there was no way they could beat the illness. Before she could hop on a plane, however, her grandparents had all but recovered and are still doing fine at the ages of eighty-seven and eighty-nine years old.

Above all, spiritual health is critically linked to physical health. I think most people's understanding of spirituality comes through a religious framework. People are born into a religion, but they don't automatically possess innate spirituality. People often grow into spirituality, and spirituality needs nurturing to grow.

I grew into spirituality over time, but most especially in recent years. The COVID-19 pandemic has brought me fully into an understanding that the things happening around us and to us in this very moment represent the hand of God, but also the evil that Satan brings into the world. For so many of us, the last three years have, at long last, brought us closer to one another and to God.

A Final Word

Using these strategies, you will possess the power and the strength to overcome the three villains by taking your health and other responsibilities into your own hands. I know that I have presented a grim view of the American, and the global healthcare systems, but I urge you not to discard proper healthcare in favor of shamanic and paganistic healthcare. Sure, teas and tinctures may improve your general wellbeing, but they will not overtly cure your illnesses—and neither will most pharmaceuticals.

Seek the support and wisdom of trained healthcare professionals, but do not be afraid to question or challenge them. Nobody can force anything into your body. You have the ability and the power to take accountability for your health.

I have made many statements throughout this chapter, many of which have been deemed "controversial" by a mainstream created to serve the Biopharmaceutical Complex. I urge you not to just take my word for it.

What follows are the accounts and the wisdom of other prominent healthcare professionals that embrace the Hippocratic standard that puts the patient first. Listen to what they have to say, compare it with what you hear from elsewhere, and draw your own conclusions.

I'm certain that you will find what we have to say compelling because it is written for your benefit, not for ours.

Peter A. McCullough

Chapter Two Takeaways

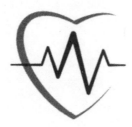

As CEO of the Wellness Company, I see that our greatest strength comes from our people, and their dogged determination to change a broken system. Therefore, having Dr. McCullough on our team, given his seniority and credentials, bolsters our strength and gives us ammunition in the battle to come.

The Biopharmaceutical Complex is a complex designed from the top down, one that requires courage to fight. It is a war—one that needs support As Dr. McCullough shows, we need to have an individual and personalized response and strategy regarding our healthcare needs. We can, as individuals, take proactive measures to take control of our health and reduce our dependence on the system. By managing our alcohol intake, our weight, and by taking personal accountability for our health, we can overcome and reject the three villains that threaten to stifle our progress against the Biopharmaceutical Complex.

In particular, we have the power to reject blind compliance to an investigative treatment that has created more problems than it solves. We can stop putting needless substances into our bodies that have the potential to do us more harm than good, and we can challenge our doctors, asking for justification behind their decisions and to see the evidence of success.

Remember, we should trust our healthcare professionals, but as in any relationship, trust must be earned. It must not be blind.

As Dr. McCullough so eloquently puts it, you are the third hero. You possess the ultimate ability and the power to fight back against the Biopharmaceutical Complex. We will help you on that journey.

Foster Coulson

Dr. Jen VanDeWater

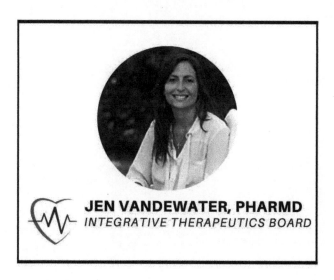

JEN VANDEWATER, PHARMD
INTEGRATIVE THERAPEUTICS BOARD

The Wellness Company's VP of Pharmacy Relationships Jen and I share a common passion: homegrown food taken directly out of our gardens, grown with love, care, and devotion. Jen has journeyed, barefoot as she will tell you, through the mire of pharmaceutical corruption at the hands of insurance giants and emerged on the other side to speak frankly and honestly about her experiences and set the path for the evolution of the relationship between the pharmacy and the doctor.

Her attitude to healthcare is simple; do what is right by the patient, not by the system that is corrupted and designed to drive high script rates and evermore expensive medications. Her attitude is to treat the patient with only what they need by understanding the patient, talking to them on the human level, and understanding their needs.

She has studied hard and understands medicines and their pharmaceutical properties acutely, and is well placed to provide the advice that she does regarding the effective treatment of COVID-19 and many other ailments that plague society today, both of the body and the spirit.

Foster Coulson

Chapter Three

The Garden is Ripe

I know both how to be abased, and I know how to abound: everywhere and in all things I am instructed both to be full and to be hungry, both to abound and to suffer need. I can do all things through Christ which strengtheneth me.

Philippians 4:13

Although I'm an Italian in New York, I'm not the kind you see portrayed on television. At four years old my parents decided to move the family from Long Island to the country because they didn't want to raise children in the city. Little did they know that some thirty-ought years later, my husband and I would be spending our free time raising chickens, tediously tapping maple sap from our own trees, and spending as much time walking barefoot in our garden as we would spend shuffling about surrounded by towering brick walls and concrete in the city. They succeeded in making me a tried and true country girl. In fact, driving through the city while visiting family in Long Island today has become quite exhausting.

My great grandparents came to the US in the early 20th Century from Italy and, as far as I know, I'm 100 percent Italian—and I wouldn't want to know otherwise. My city-dwelling cousins think it's shocking that we don't have street lights on our country roads; I just chuckle and respond, "We have headlights. Modern technology does travel outside of Manhattan and Long Island you know!" You should see them marvel at the deer coming up to my back door. You'd think we were being invaded by Sasquatch or the Abominable Snowman. "It's just a deer!"

When I was a child, my family would regularly visit us upstate for what can only be described as a feast. We'd go "hunting," as we called it. Everyone would forage for plants to eat in my parents' garden, the forest, or even from the side of the road. We'd doctor up nature with salt, pepper, and olive oil. *Mangia, mangia.*

Some of my great grandparents and other relatives deserve credit for the terrific Long Island gardens they maintained. In my family, gardening is in the blood. We were all directed to get our hands in the soil to harvest delicious, healthy meals from a young age, but it wasn't until a revealing period of time in my thirties while working as a pharmacist that I connected with my destiny to get my hands in the soil and deliver healing not just to my husband of twenty-five years now, but to the world.

My mom was incredulous earlier this year when I asked her for canning jars for my birthday instead of a dress or shoes. In my world, the Bible is the Word and that Word says, "bless the land." I suppose you could say that I'm taking the Word seriously because even before we had our garden I'd walk my property, touching the apple, pine, and maple trees as I prayed, asking God to bless my land. When 2020 rained in the terrifying news that there would be a worldwide pandemic, I added to this prayer, "...and help us survive whatever is coming."

This precious garden of mine really is something. I love getting a natural grounding by walking around barefoot in the living soil. As my happy hormones are released, I'm reminded of why children seemingly never want to wear shoes on their feet. We love sharing the sweet, vanilla-flavored maple syrup my husband labors over all day to boil down in vats over a fire with friends. We live for waking up to a cup of dandelion root coffee from our wildly grown and harvested dandelions and sip apple cider vinegar from our apple trees diluted with spring water and a touch of honey on a warm summer day. Together, we're allowing our property to live to its own full potential; its destiny is to bless us.

Recently, my husband and I packed our bags and left our Eden on a much-anticipated ten-day camping trip. We had assumed that there'd be rain, but to our surprise, there was none. Foolishly, we forgot how diligently and consistently we'd prayed in that garden of ours while rota tilling or walking barefoot in gratitude and appreciation for that symbol of our resilience, survival, and faith.

When we returned home, I struggled to look up as I walked, nervously anticipating the results of the drought in our garden. Instead, I focused on the cross my husband had made from wood and twine that hung on the fence doors of the garden. Barefoot as always, I walked through dry, yellow, and barren grass towards my beloved garden. As I opened the gate and raised my head, I was awestruck to see a miniature, living picture of what I imagine the Garden of Eden looked like. Everything was lush, green, and full of life. We had freshly ripened tomatoes, peas, and squash in abundance. God had protected our garden from drought damage. He answers prayer.

This garden is a perfect analogy of my life's story and how I came to partner with the formidable team here at The Wellness Company. Much in part due to the disturbing events of the past few years and more prominently due to the dismay I have witnessed in my work as a pharmacist for almost two decades, my values have become consecrated. Self-reliance, faith in God, and, alas, little faith in the government or Big Pharma are foundational values that compel me to bring you the story I'm about to share.

We're Escaping Slavery Out of Egypt

To the surprise of my parents, I recently asked the question, "When I was a child, did you know you were raising a David or a Joseph?" Let me give you some context as to that question.

In the Bible, David is the shepherd boy who defied the odds, picked up his sling, and defeated Goliath. Joseph, on the other hand, is the boy with the resplendent coat who was sold into Egyptian slavery by his eleven brothers only to become one of the Pharoah's officials, which led to him eventually being granted the opportunity to show his brothers mercy and forgiveness.

"Jen, you were rebellious. And in a way, we knew that would be something God would use."

And so here we are, that rebellious child who, in 2019, is heartbroken. My pharmaceutical career is not moving in the direction I once planned. In my personal prayer life, I feel like God isn't listening to me, much less answering my prayers. I explore new avenues to find a new direction as a pharmacist, possibly in local doctor's offices, but doors simply aren't opening.

Finally, I tell God that I am on the brink of hopelessness; I need a miracle.

That was the reality I faced in 2019, overwhelmed by a career that isn't offering the promise it once was; unfulfilled and empty.

That evening, I arrived at Bible study where one of the ladies chatting handed me a copy of excerpts from books that she liked. *Just what I needed*, I thought, *more words*. I was done listening to words, praying words, and reading words that simply weren't coming to life.

However, as I glanced skeptically at the paper in my hand, one quote jumped out at me.

"As a general prepares his men for battle, so have I prepared you." As I read that line, it felt like I experienced a transcendental moment; in what seemed to be an entire hour, my life flashed before my eyes. In linear time, it was probably just the blink of an eye.

I shared the story with my dad and husband, telling them that it felt as though I'd transported or left my body.

"Okay God, what is the battle you are preparing me for?" I asked eagerly, steeling myself.

At the time, I had no idea what He wanted. As He does, he sent me no immediate sign. Still, I was energized, invigorated, and a few short months later, the world changed swiftly and permanently. In the spring of 2020, I came to the realization that things around me simply didn't make sense.

Finally, I felt the Lord tell me He had prepared me for a time such as this.

The Awakening

I'm not your typical pharmacist. Much, I suppose, like I am not your typical Italian-American. I don't like to hide behind the counter. I'm a Type A extrovert who loves talking to, helping, and advising people.

In 1998 when I began my career first as a pharmacy technician, I adored the interaction and the joy of hunting down and retrieving information when people had questions. The medicine, though, didn't excite me. The pharmacists loved my gregarious and sociable nature; it gave them the opportunity to sit back and read magazines while I interacted with people. In 2006, I graduated from pharmacy college and achieved the honor of becoming a PharmD, or Doctor of Pharmacy. Math and science didn't thrill me, but the idea of working in retail and interacting with people filled me with joy.

However, from 1998 until graduation in 2006, I watched as pharmacies became robotic and autonomous, the people element eroding away. The focus became script count. When pharmacists started receiving pressure to push vaccines, an uneasy feeling grew in my heart.

Later in my career, I avoided receiving Certified Immunizer credentials; a decision that could ultimately have cost me my career.

I started my career as a pharmacist with the chain drug stores, and there, I was horrified. Everything came down to money and script counts. I was chastised for my desire to nurture and counsel people. My peers scoffed, saying, "Jen, this is a business, not a potluck."

I left the chain drug stores for a grocery chain where superiors were fairly lenient about my work because the pharmacy wasn't their primary source of profit. The pharmacy was more of an anchor for people to fill up their grocery carts. At the time, I was living in Maine where I'd been since first graduating from pharmacy college, but my husband and I felt compelled to move to upstate New York–back to our roots. Fortunately, a grocery chain there needed me, so I became licensed in New York and Vermont.

In 2010 I thought everything was going great, but the grocery chain in which I worked in Vermont shut down unexpectedly, and redundancy was on the cards. At that moment, I did not realize my professional career was about to hit a ten-year transformation.

My interview with CVS pharmacy went great, and as I gushed about loving people and helping customers understand their medications and proper usage, the interviewer told me that I was exactly what they were looking for. Apparently, they must have been desperate to fill the position, because nothing I stated in my interview up to that point was even remotely along the lines of what they wanted. In fact, although it takes more than fifteen minutes to fill a script, I was directed to tell customers that they'd never wait more than fifteen minutes. I was trained to lie to my customers, which added to the myriad of red flags I began to see.

Even more frighteningly, computers tracked everything we did. We lived in an oppressive fear of missteps; this micromanagement gave me a sour feeling in my stomach; like I was being watched and something or someone was waiting impatiently to attack or reprimand me if I messed anything up. For the next few years, I transitioned through jobs hoping to find where I belonged. I migrated from place to place, only ending more horrified than when I'd arrived.

In the chaos of my restless job hunting and mounting misgivings, I recall another moment that felt like a time-lapse or revelation. This time, I was packaging lots of fifteen or twenty pills that people were taking–sometimes up to four times a day. It felt dirty; prosaic as it sounds, I felt like a drug dealer. Here I was, facilitating the most unhealthy people in the community. They had the most medications, the most comorbidities, and the most chronic problems. It felt like I was enabling them, not healing them. Simultaneously, the community members on the least amount of medications were still long-distance running into their 90s.

I'd been trained to associate quality of life with increased prescriptions since I was in pharmacy college. Over the years, however, I never actually saw that equation add up. My colleagues shrugged it off, saying, "That's how it is, Jen. Some people are just unhealthy. They probably had McDonald's for breakfast."

There was always an excuse, but my discernment told me that I was participating in something dark. Something that was perhaps even orchestrated to promote pharmaceutical dependency. Imagine that.

Early on in my career, I was braver, perhaps–before the system just simply dragged me down. Once, while working at a grocery chain, a patient arrived, came to the drop-off counter, and reluctantly handed me her prescription. Noting her demeanor, I asked her if she was okay.

She responded by describing how her doctor had prescribed an antidepressant without discussing it much with her. She was unsure what the prescription was for, but she was dutifully fulfilling it "because her doctor told her to." As you have read in this book from Dr. McCullough and Dr. Gessling, among our absolute foundational values at The Wellness Company are personal responsibility and personal health advocacy. Question your doctor. Question the recommendations or the prescriptions that they write. Question the medications' safety.

This young woman wasn't empowered, and she certainly wasn't in the right place to make a decision about chemicals that could potentially perpetuate the pain she was feeling by masking them.

"What's going on in your life?" I asked. She told me about a challenging divorce, one that had ravaged her mental health.

I broke protocol and said, "Well look, you have a year to fill this prescription. If you take some time to process what you're going through and still want it, just let me know."

Now, truly embodying my rebellious nature, I had the audacity to sit and talk with the woman as work backed up in the pharmacy. For that moment, I found the courage to ignore the world and allow the person in front of me to feel seen and heard. In faith, I guided her both by listening to her and offering her some practical and well-intentioned advice. Having been seen as a child of God that day, her entire demeanor shifted. Her posture even shifted. Arriving with her shoulders down and face drawn, she left confident, taller, and assured that she could handle that season of her life. That was the day that I resolved to not become a pill-pusher; even though I'd have been fired on the spot if my district manager had come in during my act of rebellion.

The Tipping Point

When I'm speaking at events, people regularly approach me and ask why their doctors have changed them, for instance, from one drug to a more expensive one. It happens with everything from inhalers to heart medications. The tipping point in my pharmaceutical career; what really illustrated to me that I was working for insurance companies instead of the patients, was when I realized that those insurance companies were directing pharmacists to advise prescribers to change patient medications with no consultation between the doctors and their patients. Today, and for years before now, the direction coming down from the insurance companies to the pharmacists is to replace patients' medication with the highest "pay-out" version possible, when they can get away with it. Because doctors generally trust pharmacists, insurance companies invariably get away with this more often than not.

Doctors assume pharmacists have completed their due diligence. Doctors are simply unaware that the direction is coming from corporations and not pharmacists. Pharmacists work within their own corporate structures within which they are directed to follow orders. In short, insurance companies are making *medical decisions* for patients by commandeering prescription decisions that should be made by doctors.

Doctors are often unaware of who pulls the strings behind the chain of command; they generally don't realize that decisions are being forced upon these pharmacists to serve the financial goals of the insurance companies. Your doctor is being directed by the pharmacists as to which medication he or she prescribes; that too comes down from the insurance companies. If, say, your inhaler is changed from ABC Company to the prohibitively expensive XYZ Company inhaler, you won't be consulted; the pharmacist will simply start filling your inhaler prescription with the inhaler or medication that they've been directed to fill.

The tipping point in my career came from a phenomenon called Medication Therapy Management (MTM) that started to gradually creep into my practice in about 2010. If you think the fear of a district manager looking over your shoulder has the potential to make you sweat, you won't believe what I'm about to share with you.

Not only are pharmacists often micromanaged by district managers in the case of chain pharmacies or grocery stores, but there is another, more ominous figure that hangs over our shoulders that makes the micromanagement of district managers look like a walk in the park. That foreboding figure is much bigger, much darker, and far less concerned about individual patient needs and concerns.

This enemy is the insurance companies. Their weapon of choice with regards to pharmacies is MTM.

MTM is sold to the public as a free, one-on-one consultation with a dedicated pharmacist at a contracted MTM center. The pharmacist completes a chart review with you, asking questions about your compliance. People are enticed to participate in MTM with promises that they can save money on out-of-pocket prescription drug costs. Although MTM is commonly associated with Medicare, it has permeated all demographics in the undertaking of pharmaceutical decisions.

In almost every one of my experiences with MTM, after reviewing a patient's med chart I was directed to advise the patient's doctor to increase medications and up the dosages. Possessing an innate moral fortitude, I began performing duties that were in direct opposition to what MTM was designed for; to keep people dependent on drugs. Ideally, expensive ones.

When I started working in Long-Term Care with geriatric patients, I couldn't stomach what MTM was doing to people's bodies and wallets.

I would routinely take a family into a room and say things like, "Look, Jane, your mom is on a high-dose cholesterol medication and she's 85. Do you know why that is?"

I would empower the families to ask questions by Socratically asking them questions. Often, they had been asking these questions, too, but they thought "we" had everything under control when we filled medications for Mom that required her to throw back three cocktails of twenty pills every day. Meanwhile, Mom is a 95lb octogenarian eating like a bird. She probably had high cholesterol in her 50s when she was on more of a steak and potatoes diet. But now, thirty years later, nobody has taken the time to reduce Mom's meds. Nobody is stepping in.

To further confound this scenario, the doctors assume that the medication lowers Mom's cholesterol, so they may genuinely feel that the medication is necessary. But until the pharmacist, family, and doctor begin asking these questions, the patient will continue on the course that the insurance companies designate for them through manipulative practices that include MTM.

Families I began having this conversation with in 2016 would regularly say, "You know what, I've questioned this myself." I would then recommend that the patient goes to the cardiologist with that loved one and request that there be a review of the medication to be sure it is at the proper dosage. I personally was not able to call the doctor, I was, however, able to inspire the patient to take personal responsibility for their own health and medications. It seemed like my technical role as a pharmacist was to keep people on high doses and lots of medications.

In my heart, I knew that was wrong. I learned how to carefully provide my patients with empowering language that would enable them to request information from their physicians or specialist doctors. In this case, the family would ask the cardiologist why Mom is on such high-dose cholesterol medication. I was walking a fine line between keeping my heart aligned and keeping my job.

Upside Down Pharmaceutical Economies

What we have in pharmacies today, facilitated by MTM, is an inverted and downright perverted system of supply and demand. The model most pharmacists in America adhere to is profit over care. A pharmacist like myself didn't enter the industry - paying my way through college - to work for an insurance company's bottom line. Interestingly, when my colleagues at a previous organization that organized doctors and I conducted an exhaustive audit, we found that in the entire United States of America, there were only approximately two thousand pharmacies that filled FDA-approved medications such as ivermectin and hydroxychloroquine specifically and intentionally to treat COVID-19, although approximately eighteen thousand additional pharmacies prescribed ivermectin and hydroxychloroquine as a part of other health maintenance for patients.

You may not have any idea of how hard independent pharmacies have been hit. In 2020, there were about fifty thousand independent pharmacies across America. Since 2020, approximately ten thousand of those pharmacies have closed, maybe more. This is in part because the chain and retail pharmacies are taking over. The other part is that they cannot afford the audits that came when some of them filled safe, FDA-approved medications such as hydroxychloroquine and ivermectin; presumably saving hundreds of thousands of lives during the pandemic.

My colleagues and I at The Wellness Company adhere to supporting a healthy healthcare industry by supporting those two thousand brave pharmacies - many of them family-run small town businesses - and we're in the process of reaching out to each and every one of them as I write this chapter; barefoot, of course, looking forward to celebrating its completion with a prayerful walk around my magnificent, resilient garden.

The Biopharmaceutical Complex

As Dr. McCullough illustrates so eloquently in Chapter Two of this book, there is a hidden, upside-down pharmaceutical economy called the Biopharmaceutical Complex. Rather than operating under sound principles such as supply and demand, wherein the supplier meets demand, in the Biopharmaceutical Complex the demand is created by the insurance companies, not the patients or even the doctors.

Even more frighteningly, when pharmacists and doctors (some of whom are unknowing and only indirectly complicit) succumb to the demands of insurance companies rather than their own best judgments in accordance with their sacred patient-physician relationship, they are also unknowingly complicit in violating the Hippocratic principles of *informed consent* and *do no harm*. There is simply no justifying the way we allow non-medical professionals or insurance companies to direct what prescriptions and what brands are being filled for patients.

This is plainly criminal.

The upside-down economic structure in pharmacies incentivizes physicians and pharmacists to run their practices as businesses with strict adherence to numbers, sales, and KPIs created before doctors even meet with patients. In the case of COVID-19, this meant that millions of doses of the COVID-19 investigational gene-based therapy called a "vaccine" were produced before a doctor and patient ever had a consultation to determine whether or not that injection was appropriate for an individual patient. Across America today, pediatricians have been directed to make a blanket recommendation for every single healthy child to receive an investigational gene-based therapy treatment also called the COVID-19 vaccine for a virus from which they have zero quantifiable risks. It's unspeakable.

When executing MTM, insurance companies scroll through a patient's profile and disease state. Let's say the patient is diabetic and not taking cholesterol medication, as well. The insurance company will directly contact the pharmacy and say, "This patient needs a statin because they're diabetic and at risk for high cholesterol." Meanwhile, the patient's doctor never determined that the patient required a statin. The pharmacist never even recommended the statin. No medical professional recommended it; the insurance company did.

I have countless examples of insurance company corruption through MTM and the Biopharmaceutical Complex. In one such example, around 2016 I worked in a Long-Term Care pharmacy that filled medications.

One day, I received an MTM requesting that a cholesterol medication be added to a diabetic patient's regimen. At the time, I was unaware that the patient's cholesterol was actually within the normal range. Upon receiving the request, I performed the necessary due diligence and reached out to the patient's doctor, asking her what she wanted to do.

"No, the patient doesn't have high cholesterol and doesn't need to be on that medication." She told me with an air of incredulity. She had not sent through any prescription for cholesterol medicine and was perplexed that I had received an MTM request to put the patient on a statin. Now, the unfortunate reality is that every day in America, patients have medication added to their regimens because when the pharmacists make that call, doctors don't always take the time to evaluate these MTM requests.

Why? I was tickled when this doctor came back to me and said, "No, my patient doesn't need a statin." That doctor was doing her job, but it was the exception and not the rule. I cannot tell you how many times the doctors would say, "Great, fill the MTM request, fill the statin. Have a nice day," without taking the appropriate time required to look at the patient's charts and approve the decision with integrity, let alone consulting the patient. MTM commonly removes the patient entirely from the conversation. The patient doesn't get consulted. The family isn't brought into the conversation.

Now, I understand that I'm painting doctors in a negative light; but they have simply been poorly trained and even bullied by their parent corporations or insurance company relationships. My colleague Dr. Richard Amerling has created a comprehensive Medical Education course designed to help re-educate these doctors to promote health and not sickness. Ultimately, the conclusion drawn as a result of my work in the pharmaceutical industry was this: **we're not at war with the doctors. We're at war with the pharmaceutical companies.**

Insurance Company Bullying and Blood Money

Hopefully, you haven't eaten within the last hour, because this next part will make your stomach turn. Now, having received an MTM request from the insurance company for Drug A for patient XYZ, the pharmacist, with the prescriber's consent, is going to put that patient on a drug they may not need, about which they have never been consulted. If the pharmacist doesn't get the prescriber's consent for Drug A, the pharmacy will not get paid by the insurance company requesting the MTM. In essence, MTM compliance equals payment for the pharmacy. As you can see, small-time pharmacies are being bullied into filling medications people don't need, while large chains are willingly compliant in their pursuit of the bottom line.

On a day in 2011, the district manager, once again, was peering and looming over my shoulder, but it wasn't while I lovingly consulted the young woman going through her divorce. It was a fairly normal day and I was manning the counter in a chain pharmacy for whom I worked.

The district manager strolled through the side door and, seeing that there were no patients around, slammed a report down in front of me.

"You need to be filling more prescriptions!" He yelled. At that moment, I experienced the first of the transcendental moments that have shaped the path of my medical career. Anybody who knows me, and especially those with whom I work, know that I would rather send my colleagues Dr. Heather Gessling, Dr. Richard Amerling, Dr. Harvey Risch, or Dr. McCullough into any debate, or even a heated discussion. As I said, I am not your typical Italian-American; I'm not confrontational in any way.

Somehow in that moment, I defied one of my distinct personality traits, and I discovered a well of untapped bravery with which I responded to the district manager, "What do you want? You want me to make people sick?"

Before that moment, I somehow hadn't consciously connected the MTM abuse with such clarity. I suspected that there was nefarious profiteering involved. I knew that we were pushing more medicine onto patients who potentially did not need it. I had even observed that those consuming the least prescription medications were healthier, but that seemed to have obvious implications. Suddenly, my eyes and consciousness opened, and I realized that making people go from sick to sicker was a business plan.

An evil one.

God revealed to me in that moment that I wasn't meant to follow orders or fit in, I was called to stand out. My peers felt so dirty to me that I struggled to even sit down and have lunch with them; they made me sick to my core. It wasn't the bullying anymore, now it was the compliance that sickened me. I felt like I was turning in my neighbors to the Gestapo. That was it. It was time for me to stand up and walk out.

Some months later, I found a "mom and pop" pharmacy in a tiny Vermont mountain community. Although I was driving over an hour each way to work through the mountains of Vermont, often for two and a half hours during mountain blizzards, I was inspired by the wooden cabinets and the propensity of mountain folks to come in and chat leisurely about their dogs, their kids, their horses, and especially, their gardens.

For a brief time, I felt at peace with my work which made the taxing drive and the journey up to that point in my career seem worth it. I appreciated that my independent pharmacy boss in Vermont didn't force me to become a certified immunizer, which most other pharmacists were being forced to do.

As of writing this today on a warm summer's evening, but at the dawn of my purposeful, divine life's work with TWC, I've never administered a shot. Still though, in that tiny pharmacy in Vermont, I hadn't yet quite found my happy place. A fair amount of my work with independent pharmacies was still spent taking orders instead of consulting with patients or doctors. I couldn't shake the sense that I was working for the wrong team, despite my efforts to put the patients first.

The game is rigged. And it isn't in the best interest of patients.

In 2018, one final straw for me was standing in the back of a closed pharmacy environment where I briefly worked in a Long Term Care facility. I recall dumping twenty or so pills in my hand and thinking, *this is simply gross on my skin. I can't imagine what it's doing inside these poor folks' bodies.*

Then I began reflecting on the living corpses of people who were my age, in their 30s or early 40s, who were, too, on twenty-plus medications. Maybe it started with birth control for a teenage girl. Then perhaps the same girl started on antidepressants. And in twenty or twenty-five years; this beautiful human doesn't know what a sober baseline feels like. In truth, she's been in a medically altered state of consciousness since she was a minor.

Over the fifteen years I spent working in pharmacies, that oft-repeated phenomenon was among the most shocking experiences; seeing men and women my age taking as many pills as people in their 80s and 90s.

It broke my heart to wonder what they were like as children. If they were anesthetized or full of life and creativity. If they were going through the motions trying to make it another day, or if at one point they were full of wonder for life and deep connections with their friends. I wondered if they had ever been on a vacation without schlepping around half a dozen pill bottles or what sort of panic they'd be in if they forgot them at home. It felt, to me, like these folks were too young to be so dependent; to have so little self-reliance. To have no connection to a natural, abundant reservoir of resources; to be so young and, still, so reliant on chemicals and pharmaceuticals just to make it through the day. It also broke my heart to see those younger patients resembling dementia or Alzheimer's patients; unaware, unalert, and plain old *sfinito*, as my grandpa would say nodding towards us kids when we had so little energy at the end of a long day playing that anything other than bedtime would have been simply cruel.

Was I Brave Enough?

I know that my caring heart is a gift from God. I know that God compelled me to be a pharmacist for the people. I began to visualize leaving the pharmacy setting and becoming a voice for the doctors, who were, too, disempowered by the insurance companies. I wondered what would put wind in the sails of a campaign where we could lower doses of drugs, and even help people break free of the unnecessary "medication" that the insurance companies had essentially tricked them into taking. I wondered, *what would it be like if doctors stopped receiving incentives to keep society more pharmaceutically dependent?*

The question for me is the same as for all of you reading this book: am I brave enough?

Once I flew past the tipping point in 2019 and had collected all the empirical evidence about insurance company abuse, pharmacy abuse, and all the other coups designed for profit, not patients, I allowed myself to be jobless for a period.

This wasn't just uncharacteristic, it was devastating. I'm like a shark; if I stop moving I feel like I'll cease to live. In this jobless doldrum I grew restless, so I applied at innumerable pharmacies. Doors, though, kept slamming in my face. My spirit groaned as I now knew beyond any doubt that this system that is supposed to heal is hurting people; the broken pharmaceutical system is genuinely destroying lives. My spirit groaned when I saw the faces of patients in my head, especially the ones who had been taking so many drugs for so long that they simply looked like zombies, shuffling through and only vaguely reminiscent of who they once were.

I began praying and suddenly felt viscerally fearful. As I sat in my chair one evening in 2020, one hand placed over my heart and the other clenching my abdomen, I reflected on my journey and where I was headed. Another month without a paycheck looming. My heart was heavy and beating out of my chest; a battle drum, perhaps. My stomach was twisted and although I had eaten a light dinner, I felt like a big fat cat was clawing from within my abdomen. The room almost spun as I realized that I wasn't designed to go back into the pharmacy. I would never go back. But what did that mean?

I spoke aloud to God and said, "God, I'm scared. You guided me into becoming a pharmacist, You directed me to help the people, what do I do?"

The answer visualized in my mind, saying, "Jen, you should not fear the devil, but he certainly should fear you."

I was infused, energized with a bolt of power and bravery; it was coursing through my veins. I knew that I wasn't just going to slay Goliath, but every unholy demon that came near me. Darkness was no longer scary: darkness now feared me. And for good reason.

I Want to Dismantle the Big Pharma Agenda

We're back to 2020. I'm walking my property and praying. I've spent fifteen years in the pharmaceutical industry, but I have less direction in my career than when I was a teenager.

What I had was hope. Something gave me the courage to keep going. I began seeking out like-minded members in my community. I'd host rallies on Main Street to reinfuse the community with the hope I now had. My sister-in-law bought me a bullhorn and I would stand there and yell, "This is our 1776. Patriots never surrender!" I knew I had to keep people looking up; to be a disciple of hope and faith.

When the electricity of the elections died down in early 2021, my mother asked me why I couldn't find another independent mom-and-pop pharmacy to work with.

"Mom," I explained, "I don't want to one day stand before God and explain to Him that I needed money, so I didn't do what's right." I didn't settle.

In March 2021, I discovered a large organization of frontline doctors in America and was interested in my participation in their platform; one that was focused on restoring the quality of the patient-physician relationship. They had been wildly successful in educating the public about COVID-19 and eliminating unnecessary fear among patients, and especially parents. I was surprised when the assistant to the leader of the organization personally reached out to me.

"Hold on," she said, "you're a pharmacist who doesn't want people on meds? You want people in mind-body-spirit alignment? In total health?"

"Yes. The world wants sick care. I want to care for people."

"What's your endgame, Jen? What's your goal?"

"I want to dismantle the Big Pharma agenda," I blurted out. As soon as those words escaped my lips, I knew they weren't mine, but they were my destiny speaking through me. I thought, *if only my husband could have heard that.* He wouldn't have believed the clarity of those eight beautiful words. I. Want. To. Dismantle. The. Big. Pharma. Agenda.

I joined this doctors' organization as a volunteer in March 2021 and was promoted to a paid position as Pharmacist Liaison after one month, relishing the opportunity to work with supportive, patient-centered, caring doctors for the first time in my life. The biggest takeaway from my time with this organization was a simple revelation that carried eternal weight. God spoke to me and said, "Find them and unite them." So that's what I did.

Within months, I was participating in a pharmacist's chat room which grew to a hundred and seventy pharmacists at its zenith. It was like Christmas: Unity. Support. Connection… And I don't need to tell you how happy that extroverted Type A Jen was. By July 2021, four months after I started volunteering with the organization, I was promoted to Pharmacy Director.

Eliminated

On April 1, 2022, nine months after taking over the doctor organization's Pharmacy department, I was at home at my computer playing the "love frequency" in my ears while I worked; 528 Hz. I received an email from one of the organization managers requesting a call. I told her I could be free.

She said, "The head doctor is eliminating the Pharmacy department. There's no need for your services anymore."

She kept saying over and over again, "there's no need for your department anymore."

The woman told me I could be on the Pharmacy Team without pay. I actually considered it, but I decided to take the weekend off to pray.

When I prayed, I asked, "should I stay on the Pharmacy team? Or should I go? Should I leave the organization entirely?" Slowly, I felt peace. Peace with the unknown. I would leave.

We all know that God had something greater for me.

The Pharmacy Department was, indeed, entirely eliminated from this organization that month. To this day, I've never been given a clear direction or reason for the elimination of a department that had grown to three full-time pharmacists.

That organization's pharmacy team was intended to consist of brick-and-mortar clinics. However, we needed big donations to do that; it took a lot of real estate coordination and funding and, naturally, finding the pharmacists or entrepreneurs who were passionate about building an independent pharmacy vs. an Applebee's or Cheesecake Factory with their investment dollars. The organization had also intended to take a stab at Telehealth, but I understand that their program was priced out of the average American's budget, which in itself didn't align with my vision, mission, and core values of affordable, accessible healthcare for all. What's more, this organization wasn't having success finding enough doctors to staff such a program.

After pouring my soul into building a Pharmacy Department for this organization, being eliminated without an explanation or recognition for what I'd done was devastating. I had open projects. I had plans. But God's were bigger.

Dr. Heather Gessling suggested that I pour my heart and soul into something else. "Don't worry." She said. "God will provide the perfect opportunity."

In the middle of May 2022, I was walking through a Farmer's Market in upstate New York.

Amidst the hustle and bustle of people picking out their fruit and vegetables, Dr. Gessling messaged me and said, "Can you get on a Zoom call, Jen? As in right this minute? I have an opportunity you've been praying for."

Dr. Gessling introduced me to The Wellness Company, to its goals and ideals, all of which aligned so neatly with my own.

She encouraged me and said, "You're a warrior in this fight and this team wants you."

My previous organization dreamed of using pharmacists for pharmacy clinics. That organization's director wanted to unite the pharmacists with the doctors, and yet the pharmacists were given low-level administrative tasks to keep them busy. Astonishingly, in this period I only had five conversations and three phone calls with the Director, in over a year. We were doing things, but it wasn't moving the needle. We were treading water; we were pushing pencils.

One reason organizations that start with good intentions suffer is that, like so many startups, they don't have a clear vision. I struggled with the previous organization to execute projects because of those moving targets. It felt like we had big ideas, but after two or three weeks of heading in one direction, the course would change. The project would be left in purgatory, lingering. Some of the organizations mentioned in this book never carried their visions further than the whiteboard.

Although I was eliminated from that organization, their website eventually went live… with my face on it and claims of their intention to build pharmacies; although I understand that department was never re-established.

Dr. Richard Amerling also resigned from that doctors' organization shortly before my own elimination. In May 2022, I reached out to him. I had a list of two thousand pharmacies that my ten volunteers had worked on tirelessly for a year. I asked Dr. Amerling if he knew how I could use that list.

"Yes, Jen. I do," he replied enthusiastically. He continued to tell me about a project he was working on, but that it was very preliminary.

"Is that the same project Heather is working on?" I asked.

"Yes-" he replied

"I'm already in," I told him, barely missing a beat.

"Jen, I'm not surprised. I'm ready to move to an organization that actually accomplishes something." They say you can hear a smile through the phone; I certainly heard his.

When Heather brought me in to meet Foster for my first meeting with him, I told him about the previous organization's project and my dream of a freedom pharmacy.

"Whoa, she got rid of your department?! That idea is brilliant!"

At last, I'd finally found somebody who didn't simply want to have a great website image, but who wanted to truly help patients. With The Wellness Company, I found a home.

How Do We Defeat Big Pharma Once and For All?

Our CEO Foster Coulson, who isn't known for his hesitancy, made me VP of Pharmacy at TWC in what felt like a split second. Our leader is, if nothing else, deeply intuitive and he trusts his friends. So today, after a dark, unsettled, and tumultuous fifteen years, I get to live my vision of creating freedom pharmacies. Although big chains like CVS and Walgreens are trying to squash independent pharmacies like the two thousand we located while I worked with the previous organization, my job is to support them.

You may be asking the obvious question: "is Big Pharma too big to fail?"

In a year, absolutely yes. But gradually, residually chipped away at over time...?

This effort is going to be grassroots. People have to stop spending money at the Big Pharma locations, paying into the pockets of the insurance companies.

When you pay your insurance, you're paying Big Pharma. If you can afford to pay cash to break free of Big Pharma's grip; that's one place to start.

Support independent pharmacies. When a patient walks into a CVS pharmacy with Caremark insurance, CVS can, in many instances, be reimbursed ten times the amount the independent pharmacy would. In my time with independent pharmacies, there were times we had to turn patients away because to fill a prescription we would lose three hundred dollars. We would have to send them to the chains.

Big Pharma has tentacles in everything. More accurately, it's the leviathan. Without unity, we won't slay the beast.

Your Action Plan

Justifiably, you are surely thinking *how do we start to fight back against such an entity?* Allow me to help with that:

1. **Vote With Your Dollars.** Our first order of business is to start voting with our dollars. Again, start paying cash at independent pharmacies whenever possible. If you don't, they will go away, disappearing from our high streets and street corners. What happens when you're marked in a system as unvaccinated, and the insurance companies rule that you can't get an antibiotic or diabetes medication until you comply? Guess what, we know what will happen. Either you comply, or you die. That's why we absolutely must fight to keep independent pharmacies in business, not just surviving, but thriving.

2. **Use Virtual Doctors.** Use TWC's virtual doctors, our telehealth service. Our virtual doctors will refer you to independent pharmacies that join our network. You'll find partners both locally and virtually who will take the time to walk you through your well plan versus your sick plan.

3. **Find a Wellness Pharmacy near you.** We're now working on building Wellness Pharmacies so that awakened patients will have more independent pharmacy options near them.

4. **Become a Wellness Pharmacy owner.** Now, awakened entrepreneurs, holistic health fanatics, and even pharmacists can collaborate with us in a specialized franchise partnership. Unlike Health Mart, Good Neighbor, and Medicine Shoppe, we will never get into bed with Big Pharma.

5. **Become a fractional franchise owner.** If you're a pharmacy owner, I encourage you to become a fractional franchise owner. Host a Wellness Company supplement stand in your pharmacy. This model is like Starbucks in the grocery store. Pretty ubiquitous, eh? That's our goal. We need your support to hit it and to grow awareness of the fight against Big Pharma.

6. **Contact me for support.** If you're a pharmacist, there are creative ways behind-the-scenes to operate your business profitably and, most importantly, with more integrity. Rules and regulations change almost daily, so contact me directly to learn more. As I've said, I'm always happy to just talk to people; it's what I do. https://www.twc.health/pages/contact

7. **Share.** Ultimately, we are here to partner with you so that you can stay in business if you're a pharmacy owner or so that you can patronize pharmacies with higher vibrations if you're a patient. The goal of The Wellness Company is patient-focused care. We need it as much in pharmacies as in the clinical setting. That's why I need you to share www.twc.health with everybody

you can. We have armies of intelligent health and wellness professionals here to support everything from your gut health to your entrepreneurial whims as a partner with TWC. Join our mailing list and you'll be first to hear of every victory we achieve as we work to dismantle the system that's keeping people sick. Head over to Telegram, Signal, Truth, Gettr, Facebook, LinkedIn, or anywhere else you have a community of awakened friends and followers, and make sure they join us. Let's make TWC an army of such critical mass that Big Pharma will finally lose its stranglehold on our bodies and our pocketbooks.

Pass Down the Recipes

The final request I have for you today is to take a lesson from my grandma and *Zizis* (that's Italian for Aunt) and start passing down the recipes. My grandmother shared recipes that she learned from her grandmother, and my mother and aunts passed them down to me.

Today, people can hardly take care of their own papercuts. I'll repeat the sentiments of my friend and colleague Dr. McCullough when I tell you this: please become more health-self-reliant. God has given us these bodies as a divine gift and you've also been given the brains within your head to figure out a whole lot more than you give yourself credit for. God gave us minds and the power to use those minds, and you don't have to rely on the government, the pharmacists, your doctor, or even your pastor.

Our goal with TWC is that you will no longer make an expensive and lonely trip to the doctor every time you have an itch on your elbow. We want you to become educated and empowered enough to take care of yourself in a preventative way before you get sick. Our supplements are designed to keep your body healthy. When your body is healthy, you think more clearly, and when you're thinking clearly, you have more connection to your Source or Spirit. Your health isn't just wealth, it's a bridge to higher spiritual consciousness. When you connect to something bigger, something that empowers you, that's when life has purpose. That's when you keep getting back up when doors slam in your face.

Just eighteen months ago I pondered waitressing. I knew I'd be a terrible waitress on so many levels. I'm clumsy and I'm Italian; I can't help but stick my finger in the sauces and taste everything in the kitchen. But today, I'm here because I kept my body healthy, my mind clear, and my heart armored with hope in an otherwise dark world.

There is a reason and a purpose for your existence. It doesn't have to be in a church pew. You can hear the voice of God while sitting in the woods on a log or combing a beach at sunrise. If you're like so many Americans, you may need to find that connection in the few brief moments before dropping off your child at school and dashing to your office to get to a morning meeting, or in the few minutes you can steal in the bathroom where hopefully you're not habitually being interrupted.

If you feel caught up in the busyness and bustle of life, please take a moment today to do some deep breathing. A friend of mine religiously falls asleep to healing musical tones, whilst a colleague simply finds sixty seconds before bed to perform deep belly breathing.

When I consider that you, like me, may feel lost, my heart breaks for you.

But, you are not alone. For many of us, drugs have anesthetized us rather than empowered us. Our spirits have been numbed in many ways through alcohol, food, porn, and, yes, both legal and illegal drugs. Are you on so much medication that it's inhibiting your connection to God or the Source? Are you tired of the sensationalism from both Left and Right, vaccinated and unvaccinated, that's all fueling fear, not feeding love?

When I first began working in pharmacies, my goals were to encourage and motivate people on how to stay healthy, have great interactions with my patients, and be connected to the community. That hasn't changed, I am still *The People's Pharmacist*. Being relatable, educated, approachable, and upfront with people is part of my design. Today, I stand for the empowerment of individualized health and wellness by equipping people with the necessary tools. Head to www.TWC.health and click around. I trust your healthcare provider, your friends, your support system, or maybe even your new colleagues are there, waiting for you. I look forward to joining forces and continuing this fight. Thank you for giving me a reason to be brave. Let's be brave together, one team, an unstoppable force for a healthier tomorrow. The garden is ripe, let's pick it together.

Chapter Three Takeaways

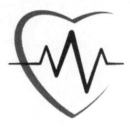

Jen's mission, along with her team at The Wellness Company is to promote the growth of strong Wellness Pharmacies throughout the US, chipping away at the bottom line of chain pharmacies and their insurance company overlords.

She has witnessed firsthand the direct impact that the corporate players in the Biopharmaceutical Complex have on the relationship between doctors and pharmacists, and how they undermine the relationship that patients have with their trusted healthcare providers by prescribing unnecessary and unwanted medications without consulting doctors or providing sound reasoning.

Jen was ahead of her time. She saw corruption very early on in her career and rejected it. Through The Wellness Company, she has found the platform she has craved to allow her to enact the change that she knows the system requires.

This is the system that works for the benefit of the patient by allowing the pharmacist the time and the energy to engage with patients on the human level, understanding their needs and, most importantly, their values and their concerns.

Prescription drug rates are, at the time of writing, 2.56 times those of other developed nations on average. This is, as Dr. VanDeWater has explained, due to a Complex that is geared towards profit and the consumption of unnecessary drugs. And this rate is continuing to grow.

By using local pharmacies, and rejecting chain and grocery store pharmacies, we can overcome the debacle that is crippling families all over the country and causing them to turn to corrupt insurance companies in an effort to gain access to healthcare that constitutes one of our basic human rights.

Foster Coulson

Dr. Harvey Risch

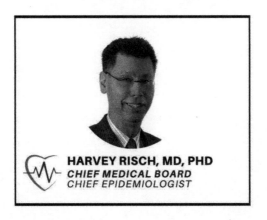

HARVEY RISCH, MD, PHD
CHIEF MEDICAL BOARD
CHIEF EPIDEMIOLOGIST

Science, or rather, good, honest, and replicable science - is one of the cornerstones of a healthy and effective medical system. For that kind of science to thrive, we need the right kind of scientists. Dr. Harvey Risch is one such scientist.

He is a man that prides himself on honesty, caught in a cherry-picked scientific community where dishonesty is rife. That is why he is so essential to the team here at The Wellness Company. We live in a world where opinion is presented as fact, distorting the overall message and impact of good science. People like Dr. Risch allow us to make the informed choices that make it possible for us to cast aside the bad science and accept that which speaks truth despite the desires of popular opinion.

In a world where common sense is cast as misinformation, Dr. Harvey Risch and those like him are instrumental in getting the right through to those that need to hear it. To amplify that message, he has taken a stand, appearing regularly on your TV screens, in your ears, and in print.

I urge you to take note as he debunks the impersonal approach of Evidence-Based Medicine, preferring instead to use scientific approaches to provide healthcare practices that truly work on the individual level.

Foster Coulson

Chapter Four

Because of Science, We Can Be Brave

"The case against science is straightforward: much of the scientific literature, perhaps half, may simply be untrue. Afflicted by studies with small sample sizes, tiny effects, invalid exploratory analyses, and flagrant conflicts of interest, together with an obsession for pursuing fashionable trends of dubious importance, science has taken a turn towards darkness."

Dr. Richard Horton
Editor-In-Chief of the Lancet

"Thank you for your bravery..." Tucker Carlson said while closing out our three-minute on-air segment this morning, just minutes before I sat down to pen this chapter at my home office in Connecticut on a July day; the stifling kind where you long for cool night breezes. I'm relieved to remove my jacket and sit back in an air-conditioned office, reflecting on the conversation with Carlson. Something feels off every time I hear it: that word bravery directed towards me. Don't kick me out of the book, but I must admit that while I appreciated the newscaster's remarks and the honest accolades of others in regard to bravery or courage, it doesn't feel quite authentic to me to accept them.

I'm proud of my role as a scientist; I've been one from the time I was maybe three years old; I have evidence to prove it. My mother recalls that I'd see the ornate cornerstone brick on a building, or I'd observe a spatula and ask, "What is this called? How does it work?"

I asked these questions incessantly, not just as a curious toddler, but until I left for Caltech in Pasadena, California for my undergrad. There, the prevailing ethos was, "I wonder what would happen if …" before figuring out how to answer that question. Indeed, I'm proud to have been a scientist since I had words to ask questions.

But brave? I'm not brave for what I have done over the past two years. I'm… well… authentic. To be honest, I would say I'm stubborn in my scientific beliefs. If I get something wrong, I'll update my beliefs in accordance with new knowledge. But until I consult with science, I keep my mouth shut, which often eliminates the need for me to eat my words. You see, science makes it easy to tell the truth… provided you're not putting propaganda in Nature's mouth and calling it science. You just report what Nature tells you.

Over the past forty years, I've published approximately four hundred peer-reviewed scientific research papers which have been cited more than forty-six thousand times. My H Index is 102 at the moment, which means that 102 of my papers have been cited more than 102 times.

To say that I've had an active career in epidemiology is an understatement. It's been fruitful, but I've stood on the shoulders of giants. Among those giants are the minds of my own kin; my father a clinical psychologist and my brother Neil, always having been brilliant, now a Statistical Geneticist at UC San Francisco. He's also past President of the American Society of Human Genetics. My first cousin Robert (Bobby) Risch has a mathematical algorithm named for him and is a retired mathematician at IBM. As a kid I used to prowl the neighborhood for discarded TVs, and having learned to solder at age eleven, I had fun taking them apart in order to use their parts to make other electronic devices. Science is in my genes, in my very nature.

In 1957, Sputnik happened and, unlike today, society turned to collectively push and promote science education on everybody: creating opportunities for scientific education at all grade levels in a much stronger way than in the generation before. Sputnik led the United States to enact concerted reforms in science and engineering education due to the threat that the Soviets would out-engineer us. On the one hand, the reforms were a response to the embarrassment that the Soviets had outpaced us in rocket technology. On the other more urgent hand, Sputnik illustrated that the Soviets possessed technology that could launch nuclear bombs at us. This elicited more hands-on laboratory elements in the classroom as well as the input of scientists who previously hadn't enjoyed a say in academic curriculum design.

Propelled by my thirst to understand the way the world works - an element of my character that has only become more concrete over the decades and supported by the encouragement of my scientifically-minded family and education - I began exploring a variety of concentrations during my undergrad.

By any standard, I have had about the best scientific education on the planet. From the time I entered Caltech, I became personally acquainted with several Nobel laureates. My advisor was Ed Lewis, who received the Nobel Prize in Biology after I left. I had several interactions with the physicist Richard Feynman and took a course with Roger Sperry, the neuropsychologist who earned a Nobel Prize in Physiology and Medicine in 1981 for his discoveries concerning the functional specialization of the hemispheres of the brain. At Caltech, the introductory classes were not taught by junior faculty making their way up the academic ladder, but by the most senior professors with solid international reputations.

In medical school, my professors included Elizabeth Barrett-Conner, who impressed me with her profound knowledge of cardiovascular epidemiology. My pathology preceptor was Dr. Averill Liebow, who had come from Yale and had been a fellow under Milton Winternitz, the revolutionary 1920s Dean of Yale Medical School. Winternitz was a demanding, imposing figure to train under.

Without a doubt, the quality of those professors rigorously informed my scientific outlook. In my Ph.D. work at the University of Chicago, I learned biostatistics from Paul Meier of the Kaplan-Meier method for survival analysis. For my Ph.D. dissertation, I worked on a difficult mathematical model of infectious epidemics and later published some of that work.

Finally, after graduate school, I completed a postdoctoral fellowship at the University of Washington, which has been one of the primary epicenters of cancer epidemiology research in the world. I learned epidemiology under Professor Noel Weiss and biostatistics under Professor Norman Breslow.

I then moved for my first job at the University of Toronto, where I learned hands-on epidemiologic field methods to gather experience in carrying out these kinds of research studies in the population, under the tutelage of Dr. Anthony Miller. Maybe you could say that I was in school for too long, but I would argue that all of this education satisfied some of my scientific curiosity. It's hard to create a more comprehensive preparation for one in science, and those mentors and professors brought me to where we are today and toward the future we are creating with urgency and vigor following the scientific heresies of the past two years.

From that chaos, we will seek order.

What Happens When a Jet Plane Engineer, A Psychologist, and An Epidemiologist Walk into A Bar?

As I said, I got my Ph.D. in the mathematical modeling of infectious epidemics and then moved to postdoctoral work and a career in cancer epidemiology research. Thirty years later, I was elected to membership in the Connecticut Academy of Science and Engineering. When the COVID-19 pandemic led to widespread lockdowns, the Academy decided to create an additional advisory committee to help the governor figure out how to get out of a lockdown; we were tasked with thinking outside the box.

So, there we were, a committee that included a jet-plane engineer who understood how to manage air motion, a clinical psychologist who understood how to manage human behavior, and a plethora of interesting people across a multitude of disciplines collaborating on a strange new public health committee.

I was tasked with evaluating early treatment, so I studied the literature. In April 2020, I began making observations about medications that were being used and those that weren't. I wrote an extensive paper in the American Journal of Epidemiology that was peer-reviewed by the editors of the journal. The report identified strong evidence across five studies that the malaria/arthritis medication hydroxychloroquine, when used as part of a multidrug regimen starting in the first five days of treatment for COVID-19, elicited success for almost everybody treated. You might say that the rest was history.

My findings garnered heavy attention in the media and, as you've probably heard, a little unscientific pushback from some academic circles. I simply credit my supposed bravery with the phenomenon of being in the right place at the right time and reporting objectively and stubbornly about the evidence. Science after all, when conducted right, does not lie. That right place was at the confluence of science and a public health emergency where I had the honor (or maybe naïveté) of speaking the truth. In war, the first casualty is truth. My rank as a senior epidemiologist and my having the weapon of accurate science have allowed me to lead some troops effectively, and as you'll read towards the end of this chapter; even save some lives.

As a rule, I simply use evidence as my guide. In some respects, I suppose that's what has helped my message gain traction. It's not a message per se, but the science that people craved in an environment riddled with misinformation and marketing objectives where peoples' lives were at stake. From April 2020, my observation was simply this: we need not fear this virus when early treatment is proving powerful and effective—objectively and empirically. Whether a drug works for a treatment or not is a fact of nature.

I'm not interested in the senseless opining on social media from people who are not qualified to come to conclusions about things they don't fully understand. I don't do social media and was only reluctantly compelled to start a Telegram channel simply to make sure that people interested in following my media appearances or published articles will have access to a stream of authentic Risch materials.

We live in a natural world with both plausible explanations for how it works, as well as preposterous theories that are accurate to a hair's thickness across the width of the United States. How these laws came to be is the mystery of our existence, but what is more remarkable to me is that we humans have evolved the intellect to have figured all of this out. Regardless, while such scientific theories point us to doing scientific studies and I love the theories, I am an epidemiologist because only the empirical data in groups of people are definitive for how things work in medicine.

Our Modern-Day Sputnik

Following my paper in the American Journal of Epidemiology in May 2020 and its somewhat tepid legacy media reception, I continued to study early treatment. Despite a glimpse of adoption by the Trump Administration before his administration saw more opportunity with a vaccine for his reelection, the media began smearing hydroxychloroquine, holding its potential right up there with drinking bleach to kick COVID-19. I realized that this was a systematic media problem; an outpatient disease such as early stage COVID-19 was being misrepresented as its later hospitalized disease stage, where the immune system overreacts to the virus and fills the lungs with immune system debris. They are two separate diseases and require distinct treatments, and the media was systematically conflating the two.

Media sources sporadically allowed me the microphone to discuss early viral illness, the question of viral replication, and the immune system's ability to cope with that. However, they were unprofessionally extrapolating details of hospital disease to address outpatient disease. I relayed evidence of what my friend and colleague Dr. Zev Zelenko had successfully accomplished; treating people with hydroxychloroquine, in medication recipes to which he later added ivermectin. Among doctors following Zev's recipes are found: Dr. Peter McCullough, Dr. Brian Proctor, Dr. George Fareed, Dr. Brian Tyson, and Dr. Didier Raoult, the last of whom had independently developed similar recipes in France. What all of these doctors have in common is the ability to espouse empirical knowledge coupled with what they had gleaned from studies in the early 2000s related to chloroquine and hydroxychloroquine and SARS 1, among others. Although I wasn't a clinician, I was the scientist evaluating epidemiologic and real-world evidence gleaned from the clinicians.

Over the pandemic, various myths have persisted. Among the biggest is the obsession with the number of cases. In short, not every case of COVID-19 has been bad. As it turns out, relatively few were. COVID-19 is a spectrum of responses to a spectrum of organism strains. Cases per se do not seriously matter in this pandemic; "long Covid," hospitalizations, and mortality do. Case illness can be unpleasant, but as long as it remains outpatient and resolves on its own without long-term consequences and hospitalization, it is considered medically mild and provides a strong degree of natural immunity.

The dramatic focus on new cases and different strains have been leveraged as a tool for societal control; people that are afraid are easily manipulated. In my experience, when a respiratory virus mutates and grows in transmissibility it becomes more infectious and usually less harmful, and as a result, we see fewer people die. That is what has happened with Omicron versus the previous strains, and now with the common BA.5 strain which is generally even less serious than the original Omicron.

Today, assessing the past poor decisions of our public health officials isn't as mission-critical as addressing the holes we've uncovered in our scientific processes and establishments. Millions of people rightfully don't trust medicine, they don't trust their doctors, they don't trust public health, and they don't trust government institutions; they're wise to be so skeptical. In short, most of our American neighbors have been woefully misinformed and intentionally deceived.

The trust and appreciation one used to feel for their doctor has deteriorated, and with good reason. Doctors have been either consciously or otherwise silenced and paralyzed from looking at the very same research that has guided me over the past two years. In many cases, when doctors were conscious of the crimes, they failed to speak up because they were worried about losing their jobs. If they weren't aware of the crimes: that's a failure of our systems in education, training, and accountability.

Rather than blasting on the news that telemedicine groups have successfully treated more than a quarter of a million Americans with drugs that we're not allowed to talk about, and rather than supporting an environment of healing, we've perpetuated death either through ignorance or the reluctance to examine empirical evidence. At the risk of sounding calloused, I assure you there's a silver lining. And if you're still reading, I suspect you're a part of the much-needed reform to our medical systems, policy, and, alas, suppression and censorship of truth-wielding scientists like the ones you're reading about in this book.

This is our modern-day Sputnik revolution.

Whispers of Corruption

As my colleagues Dr. Jen VanDeWater and Dr. Peter McCullough have clearly illustrated, something fishy is going on. Pharma corruption in medicine is everywhere and the legacy media is functionally paid as agents of pharma. The massive amount of direct-to-consumer advertising of pharma products across the legacy media as well as in medical journals has addicted those companies to the Pharma-controlled income.

It's difficult to get objective voices into the mainstream narrative. I'm lucky enough to be one of the few medical scientists who doesn't operate through pharma grants. I'm not allegiant to Pharma and, most likely, they would never give me a grant now. There's a problem with the public not knowing what to believe because of the Pharma influence on our media. Happily, many people have found their way to alternative medical care systems.

Because primary care doctors were either too fearful to meet with patients in person when they had outpatient COVID-19 or because they were simply too lazy or stubborn to find out what was working with other doctors who were successfully treating patients, people were told to stay at home, drink liquids, take Tylenol, and go to the ER if they couldn't breathe. Because of the corporate ownership of many practices, doctors didn't feel like they could go off protocol because instead of exercising the independent expert authority they have to take care of patients, they're worried about kowtowing to bosses in a corporate environment. In America today, corporations make many medical decisions, not doctors.

This is the reason that you're reading this today. It's high time that we break free from the corrupt corporate control of medicine. If you weren't already royally incensed, you've at least had a funny feeling that things are somehow "off" with regard to our medical system.

When I went to medical school in the mid-1970s, my classmates and I were already aware of this corruption. Even fifty years ago we didn't want to take books from drug companies. We didn't want the free stethoscopes and doctors' swag bags. These blandishments turned into obligations.

Pharma has, for a very long time now, spent more on marketing than drug development. Six billion dollars, which is what Pharma spends on advertising, goes way further than putting ads on TV, newspapers, and magazines. Six billion dollars of ads don't just get public exposure mileage for the drugs in question, but it also generates allegiance from the media. That media platform doesn't want to lose this vast income from

Big Pharma, and in some cases, they simply can't. Media is dependent upon Big Pharma money. It's consistent, it's reliable, and it's substantial. Media is in many ways being controlled by that steady income stream and the sources of that income.

The Case for Telehealth

My colleagues aren't happy with being told how to practice medicine, and that's why I believe a company like TWC, with whom I've partnered, is exemplary. The doctors I'm working with are passionate about being able to use their best judgment and take care of patients without the micromanaging of hospital bosses or generic protocols overshadowing honest conversations and collaborations with patients. These TWC clinicians will not settle.

Just think about it: how can a patient get a second opinion if all doctors have to comply with uniform treatment protocols? Medicine is not an exact science and expert experienced judgment is one of the most important characteristics of a good doctor. Where is that, if everything is cookie-cutter? You might as well get medical care from a checklist.

Today in the US, there are many active telemedicine groups. In fact, one colleague shared with me in late July 2022 that his group has treated more than 275,000 Covid patients over the past two years—with only six deaths.

That is proper medical care.
This is what we're striving for.

The ability to treat patients with our best scientific medical knowledge.

TWC's virtual doctors and video telemedicine is among many brave initiatives in this space. As a fair warning, some telemedicine groups are not managed and operated by teams of medical freedom fighters; some of them have, indeed, formed allegiances with drug companies, and some are just email services for writing prescriptions and never actually see their patients. When exploring telemedicine groups, as with anything: do your diligence. Telehealth is a growing segment of the healthcare industry that isn't just worthy of notice but celebrates a physician's freedom to treat patients with the best scientific and medical knowledge.

Medicine has evolved tremendously over the past thousand years, but it's truly transformed over the past two hundred years with a scientific era of Western thought. We've amassed a huge amount of medical knowledge. Really very little of this was gained through randomized trials, but we didn't exactly kill all of our patients with medications that didn't work, either. Doctors, over hundreds of years, used educated guesswork and passed their successes on to future generations, and medical knowledge accumulated with monumental velocity this way.

Today, I imagine that approximately eighty to eighty-five percent of drugs are used off-label from how they were originally approved. Dr. Gessling suspects that number is at least seventy percent. This is an example of medical independence and the free ability to find the best solutions for each patient.

Doctors do not need randomized trials to prove everything in order to have medical validity. Despite Dr. Fauci's dismissive remarks calling real-world evidence "anecdotal," by which he means "junk science," the accumulated scientific evidence in medicine is not anecdotal. It's the result of centuries of medical independence.

There are several paths to obtaining medical evidence. Randomized trials, non-randomized controlled trials, clinical evidence, and epidemiologic evidence all help us understand sickness and wellness. A case series of fifty, a hundred, or even five hundred cases isn't anecdotal. It is real scientific evidence of its own kind. It deserves to be taken apart and understood the way that science does.

Dr. Heather Gessling modeled scientific integrity when she began traveling around the country to speak with other doctors at conferences, looking for answers to why her patients were not responding to treatments that had previously worked well. Testing, sharing notes, recalibrating treatments, and achieving results that save lives is a model for how to provide quality medical care; doing our best to minimize harm as much as we can, and doing our best to be right as much as we can without the medical straitjacket of corporate medicine telling doctors to blindly follow orders and recreate the recipe prescribed for every patient, no matter what. Most of the time the decrees from corporate medicine will be approximately wrong; sometimes they will be catastrophically wrong.

And so, we're left with a strong case for telehealth. Telehealth allows doctors to practice with a degree of medical integrity, free of the corporate straitjacket, without the distraction and overhead of retail space. It's a significant advancement in medicine, whether the public is consciously aware or not.

Telehealth is already being used by between twenty-one and twenty-six percent of Americans among most demographic subgroups, a number that is lower among the uninsured (9.4 percent) and young adults (eighteen percent.) Black individuals and those with Medicaid and Medicare take advantage of telehealth at rates of twenty-seven percent, twenty-nine percent, and twenty-seven percent, respectively. Among those earning less than twenty-five thousand dollars annually, twenty-seven percent use telehealth.

Telehealth will not on its own be a substitute for physical examinations and medical procedures, but it can provide an important first line of primary care that can treat many common conditions, as well as refer patients for laboratory, x-ray, or ultrasound testing, and as indicated, to an in-person office or hospital visit. Its convenience and popularity already show that it works extremely well for a substantial part of medical care in addition to psychological or psychiatric care.

When I was a child, my pediatrician made house calls and provided care that was custom-tailored to me and my brother from the best of his experience, wisdom, training, and understanding of medical literature available at that moment in time. In some way, telemedicine takes us back to that unique time; it goes back to convenient, personalized care. Quality of care. The doctors with our company publicly rejected the fear-mongering and antagonistic messages on the legacy media that told the public they would die without the COVID-19 vaccine. These doctors had the tools to treat patients successfully, and many of those doctors endured a significant amount of pushback. The doctors in our company treated illnesses that the public messaging said were not treatable.

Let's say you don't live in Florida or Texas, and you don't have the opportunity to find the care and treatment that has been suppressed in so many other states. Telemedicine opens the door for you to experience high-quality independent-thinking medical care–not regimented one-size-fits-all medical care. As a scientist, I want to see the best science as I understand it being used in medical care. I want to see the best outcome for patients, not the best outcome for corporate profits. If the science is better, the doctors will be better and their results will be better. That is the TWC model. And for that reason, I'm all in.

Plausibility Fraud and A Return to Scientific Education and Critical Thinking

Dr. Gessling details in Chapter One the failure of her medical education to illustrate the importance of nutrition in a patient's personal chemistry. Dr. McCullough has enlightened us about what he calls the Biopharmaceutical Complex. Dr. VanDeWater made a compelling case for a different way to interact with our doctors and subsequent pharmaceutical regimens. And now, I will take a moment to share my personal views on Plausibility Fraud and the need to return to scientific education and critical thinking.

Over the past two years, I've engaged in learning about branches of medicine that I took for granted. In medical school, my colleagues and I were trained to trust where the messages come from; essentially indoctrinated about how medicine works. You're directed to read scientific literature for as long as you practice, but I found that, by and large, most MDs fail to keep up with the very latest discoveries and advancements;

they typically receive continuing medical education through lecturers paid by drug companies.

Although I became a medical scientist rather than a clinician and haven't practiced medicine since medical school, I learned more about COVID-19 than many of my practicing clinician peers over the past two years because I invested all my time in reading and thinking about scientific papers and performing some of the original research with medical colleagues as well. This was second nature to me; it's what I've done for my entire career. So why haven't these practicing doctors? They're putting their hands on patients, and their patients trust them. That's a monumental responsibility.

What I've learned is that the messages we're being fed are based essentially on plausibility, not science. There is a huge but subtle difference. The messages come from the government and spokespeople from agencies such as the CDC, the FDA, and so on. They're feeding us plausibility, and plausibility is sneaky; it fools people because they don't know the difference. The problem is, it also fools doctors. Doctors routinely use plausibility for the reasoning behind the symptoms patients have. For instance, if your patient has a strep sore throat and you figure that out, you're not going to start making biological theories about the bacteria the patient is battling. You're not going to enroll five hundred patients with similar symptoms and five hundred without and study their differences. You already know what the cause is and how to treat it.

However, when people present with something new, something unclear, then the job is to start making biological medical theories about different pathways in an attempt to figure out a differential diagnosis. Your claim is theory until experiments are conducted in a controlled way. That's when theory becomes science. Making the theory is the motivation for science, but it isn't science. It's the plausibility part. The science comes when studies are completed to establish or refute the theory.

Theory is what has been marketed to the lay public as well as doctors. Plausibility. Plausibility, for instance, that some drug doesn't work because its concentration has to be too high. We've seen this with the case of ivermectin. The marketing messages and plausibility claims indicated that ivermectin couldn't work because it had to be too high of a concentration in the lab experiment in order for it to be effective in humans, but it turned out that that theory was incorrect in real-world use.

We've seen more. Let's take the messaging about distancing, vaccines, and virtually everything in society and public health. Our schools, businesses, and every other facet of our lives were turned upside down on the basis of plausibility. On the basis of believable messaging.

For example, the plausibility that putting a mask in front of your nose and mouth blocks things from getting through in either direction. People believe that message because it looks to the naked eye that if you put a filter in front of something, you block it. In truth, it's like putting up a chain-link fence to block mosquitoes. It just doesn't work. What we need to do is start from theories before conducting controlled experiments, drawing and disseminating conclusions from the experiments, not from the theories. Put the masks on people and see what really happens. Do the studies. Do the science.

I'm an epidemiologist, which means that my job is to do the science. I conduct controlled experiments on people to see whether things have relationships. Theories motivate us. Theories compel science. Theories may be believable, but theory is not science. Theories brainwashed the public for two years into putting masks on or labeling a previously FDA-approved medication as a horse dewormer.

There's been a huge amount of publishing both in peer-reviewed and preprint papers. There have been thousands of opinions shared based on highlights from some of these papers. And, of course, there's an undeniable drug company bias in medical media. Until people - both lay people as well as doctors - read the original papers, what we're seeing is sensationalism and misinterpretation or the embellishment of studies that, in some cases, were fatally flawed from the get-go.

My job over the last two years has been to comb through the original research papers and try to make sense of things. To think critically about them. To look over the data that's put out by the CDC and try to make sense of that. To see whether the things the CDC publishes in their Morbidity and Mortality Weekly Reports are believable, or if they're flawed.

In over forty years of teaching master's and doctoral students in epidemiology, I have taught my students to examine research papers by looking at what the authors said, what the studies actually show, what you can infer from the studies, and what the studies in the medical pieces of literature as a whole are really demonstrating. You would be surprised to see that in many instances, what authors write as the conclusions of their studies are not what the studies show. You have to study the study—to look over the paper with a suspicious mind, trying to catch inconsistencies and problems, and only when you have satisfied yourself that nothing materially problematic is there, can you accept that a study contributes to scientific knowledge. This is how proper science is done—not by reporters copying the last line of the paper's abstract.

I recently heard of a doctor with a busy Vail Valley practice in Colorado who said, "I just wish there was one place that aggregated solid, reliable interpretations, information and updates, particularly with regard to the COVID-19 vaccine and effects thereof."

Here at TWC, that's our goal; to provide solid accumulated scientific and clinical resources in one place from our Chief Medical Board, currently, the doctors who each have a chapter in this book.

However, I also cringe at something else in this altogether brave and heart-centered doctor. He's compassionate, he's eager for the truth, but he needs somebody to do the legwork for him because of how busy he is. On the one hand, he's exactly the kind of doctor we want caring for patients. On the other hand, I want him to seek evidence and understanding from the original papers as much as possible.

At TWC, that's what we want to be; a resource, but certainly not a crutch. If this brave doctor is reading my words today, I would tell him, "Please, use the resources we provide from the TWC Chief Medical Board. In addition, I would also encourage you to use your own critical reasoning. Let's work together."

Believe me, it's going to be a lot of work to restore integrity to medical messaging.

The Plausibility Failure of Evidence-Based Medicine

In Chapter Five, you'll learn about Evidence-Based Medicine, or EBM, from Dr. Richard Amerling and I believe that he has put it into terms and stories that will not only fascinate you but inspire you for what the future of medical education should look like. I'll set the stage here with a discussion about EBM.

EBM started with an idealized notion that the only thing that will tell us whether drugs work is a double-blinded, randomized controlled trial. That already was a misrepresentation that sounded plausible. Again, plausibility is sneaky. It fools lay people, but it also fools doctors. It's easy to trust a source that states, "We'll do quality work and great scientific studies to see whether medications work, whether vaccines work, and so on," but doctors and lay people are evolving. We're finding over the past two years that so many of these studies were not good because people did not recognize that randomized trials have problems just like non-randomized trials, just like other kinds of epidemiology.

Every kind of study has its good and bad parts. What has been misrepresented in EBM is that randomization automatically cures everything—it cures all the problems. That is based on a naive falsehood that has a high plausibility value, and it fails to understand epidemiology.

In epidemiology, you always have a potential third factor, called a confounder. The confounder can be the real reason behind the relationship between exposure and outcome. If so, that confounder has to be controlled or adjusted. Randomization asserts that if you randomize the people on the drugs, there cannot be confounding because everybody is balanced; the presumption is that randomization makes everybody equal except for the treatment.

The unrecognized problem is that randomization only works in very large studies when the number of people who get the disease, in both the treatment and placebo groups, is more than one hundred or so. Randomization works then because in large numbers, the differences will not be particularly large. However, in small studies with few outcomes, the differences can be proportionally large with randomization. In every randomized trial, we need to know how big the differences are.

For example, flip a coin ten times. You might get seven heads and three tails. That happens by chance. Seven heads and three tails mean that something about that coin in those ten flips was more than twice as likely to be heads as tails. Or it might be seven tails and three heads. This is just chance, but if you have seven people with a disease in the treatment group and three in the placebo group, even if it happens by chance, that's potential confounding. Now, if you have five hundred flips, you're going to get much closer to a 50/50 split between heads and tails. Randomization would work with these numbers. Simply put, in larger experiments, you will achieve more accurate results. More critically, it's easy to have distorted studies when the numbers of outcomes are small. Randomization is useless when you have a small number of outcomes, and the claim that randomization gives the study weight and validity is wrong.

That is why some of the randomized trials published in the *New England Journal of Medicine* and *The Lancet* misrepresented their importance. A study with forty thousand people does not make it a big study; it takes hundreds of outcomes to qualify as a big study.

Let's say you have a vaccine trial. In each group, you have twenty thousand participants. Perhaps the vaccine will reduce the number of infections over the study, but then you observe six hospitalizations in the vaccine group and twenty-eight in the placebo group, and the definitive assertion that the vaccine reduced the risk of hospitalization when nothing of the case is true. The numbers are way too small for that degree of difference not to have occurred by chance. When there are two deaths in one vaccine arm and one death in the other and the study is claimed to be a randomized controlled study, that's nonsense. This can actually be worse in randomized trials than in non-randomized but controlled trials. In the latter, investigators know that they have to adjust for potential confounding factors, so they measure everything that they think might be important and adjust for those factors—things like age, weight, chronic illnesses, smoking, and the like. However, in randomized trials, investigators usually think that randomization automatically prevents confounding, so they don't adjust for anything. That is a problem for randomized trials with small numbers of outcomes.

Randomized trials are designed to have enough statistical power to "see" a certain size of benefit to, say, cut mortality in half. "See" means to be able to separate the association from the random statistical noise. To be valid though, these studies also have to be able to reduce the potential confounding, but they are never designed for that. That's the plausibility failure of Evidence-Based Medicine. Largely, this plausibility failure in EBM has gone unnoticed.

Aside from me, I know of one Princeton statistician by the name of Angus Deaton who published a paper about this a few years ago. It's an important technical paper that everyone who carries out randomized trials and everyone who reviews them should read.

Confounding can occur by chance or from some systematic relationship between the variables that you measure, but once you do a study, it's either in your data or it's not. You don't get to claim a valid result without looking at the amount of imbalance of people, which is not generally taken into consideration in these EBM studies. Both doctors and the public have simply been misled about the assumed quality of the scientific results of randomized trials. In many instances, this reflects a Pharma narrative.

There are other ways that randomized trials can be corrupted or subverted: for example, ending the trial too soon, or conducting the trial in a geographic area where the placebo people can go out and buy the drug over-the-counter, which happened in a Brazilian study of ivermectin. These plausibility frauds have corrupted much of the pandemic.

My goal is to convince the general public that there is much more to science than the little bit of manipulated possibilities that have been officially proclaimed.

Fauci said, "Trust me, I am the science," but he has only talked about plausibility claims of science and not the actual science. The general public, even some people in my family and in the general public who are lay people that do not feel equipped to read the original scientific papers depend on scientists to determine the worth of those papers. If the medical scientists in the legacy media are all directly or indirectly paid agents of Pharma, sometimes receiving grants from Pharma, our media is necessarily corrupted.

The very language of science is perverted by these entangled, financially compensated, or nefariously motivated actors. Hydroxychloroquine (HCQ) and the hoopla surrounding it starting in early 2020 is an example of how one doctor, Anthony Fauci, perverted public opinion with messages that berated and dismissed the valiant efforts of Dr. Vladimir Zelenko in treating patients successfully with HCQ combined with zinc and azithromycin, later called "the Zelenko Protocol."

Zelenko heard about HCQ when investor James Todaro and lawyer Gregory Rigano tweeted links to papers showing promising results with chloroquine usage in both China and France. Unfortunately, Dr. Fauci said no. Literally. He stated, "The answer is no. The evidence that you're talking about is anecdotal… it was not done in a (randomized) controlled clinical trial, so you really can't make any definitive statement about it."

That was false. "Anecdotal" means a case report of one person, or two, potentially even three. A study of forty people is not anecdotal, it is a case series. A study of Dr. Zelenko successfully treating four hundred patients is not anecdotal, it is a major case series.

While such evidence is not as strong as a controlled trial, it is nevertheless evidence. My first COVID-19 publication, published in May 2020, was a review of all of the then-available studies of HCQ use in COVID-19 outpatients. That review, which included controlled trials, provided strong evidence that HCQ significantly reduces the risk of subsequent hospitalization and mortality in COVID-19. Since then, every further study of HCQ use starting within the first four or five days during symptoms in high-risk COVID-19 outpatients has shown significant reductions in the risk of hospitalization and mortality. This time, there were more than forty thousand patients studied across the world. Every study shows the same thing. The drug works exceedingly well. So ask yourself, why was Fauci so wrong?

By mid-2020, we had evidence that HCQ, particularly in a combination of three safe ingredients, could likely save lives. Doctors all over the country, if they had understood Fauci's lie, could have been off to treat patients who got sick. Children may have finished the school year. They may never have been put into masks. People would not have died alone in hospitals.

Even today, in hospitals across America, patients are being denied one of the most important factors in their healing: connection with others. What would have happened if Dr. Zelenko's treatment protocol had been conducted on a wider scale as opposed to, well, nothing? What are we going to do to ensure that the future holds people accountable for the perversion of messages with scientific terms, like Fauci? What would happen if next time we are united, and therefore, better prepared to call out corrupt players like Fauci? That's the world I believe we're creating with TWC.

A Fearless Future

In the future, I hope that more lay people, as well as doctors, will review original scientific studies and draw their own conclusions. A friend of mine regularly goes to NIH or PubMed online and considers this "research into the original study" because it's not the *Washington Post* or *New York Times* interpretations. This is hard, but it's what has to be done until all of the corruption in medicine has been brought out into the open and cleaned up.

The absence of evidence is not the same as evidence of absence.

There is one other reason that my heart goes out to the busy doctor in Vail who is eager for the Chief Medical Board at The Wellness Company to begin publishing our interpretations of studies. You cannot trust the conclusions of authors without careful and suspicious review. On some level, you shouldn't trust anybody but yourself, either. Even though I trust my colleagues here at TWC, I implore you to exercise your critical thinking skills daily.

When the media picks up on conclusions, especially when these conclusions are drawn for political or financial motives, science gets subverted in full public view.

Having taught epidemiology students for so long, I have discussed these problems in studies over and over again in the classroom setting, but what we have seen in the past two years is the Superbowl of the medical and scientific communities' failure. And yes, even to the extent of being nefarious and intentionally misleading.

It takes a very strong amount of psychological fortitude to resist the fear, whether it's COVID-19, Monkeypox, or some new media fear-mongering. What I would gift to you is the adherence to critical thinking. When you're grounded in science, fear tends to subside rather quickly. Surround yourself with a community that is committed to carefully reviewing original studies and, even if there is a scary outcome suggested, band together to protect one another through education. For a fearless future, we must think critically.

The next step in "Dr. Harvey's recipe" for a fearless future is one where there is free speech. The only reason to suppress or censor speech is that you do not have a compelling argument to make in rebuttal. Censorship is a tool to substitute for argument, and its use proves that the party using it has no argument. Science works only by argument and debate, not by censorship.

Science also does not work by consensus. By the time a consensus has been reached on a topic, the evidence has moved on and the consensus is almost certainly wrong. All those so-called consensus statements published over the last two years by medical specialty boards are essentially wrong. Worse, they are irrelevant.

This is because they are not science. This fact was explained in the 1950s by the well-known philosopher of science, Karl Popper, who said that statements about the beliefs of scientists have no relation to statements about the workings of Nature. For that, you have to go back to the original studies and understand them yourself.

To put this in the words of physician and writer Michael Crichton:

> *"I want to pause here and talk about this notion of consensus, and the rise of what has been called consensus science. I regard consensus science as an extremely pernicious development that ought to be stopped cold in its tracks. Historically, the claim of consensus has been the first refuge of scoundrels; it is a way to avoid debate by claiming that the matter is already settled. Whenever you hear the consensus of scientists agrees on something or other, reach for your wallet, because you're being had."*

Let's be clear: the work of science has nothing whatsoever to do with consensus. Consensus is the business of politics. Science, on the contrary, requires only one investigator who happens to be right, which means that he or she has results that are verifiable by reference to the real world. In science, a consensus is irrelevant. What is relevant is reproducible and replicable results. The greatest scientists in history are great precisely because they broke from consensus.

There is no such thing as consensus science. If it's consensus, it isn't science. If it's science, it isn't consensus. Period.

Thank You for Your Bravery

On July 1, 2022, I retired as an active professor of some forty years from Yale University and now work as Professor Emeritus as well as Senior Research Scientist. I still have research studies going on.

Over the past two years, I've received more than a hundred thousand emails from people asking me anything from, "How do I get past the vaccine mandate in my workplace?" to "Where can I get Hydroxychloroquine?" to "I have a high fever and I feel like death, what can I do to beat COVID-19 before it beats me?"

As a rule, I've answered every conceivable email that I could answer; often referring that person to a qualified doctor or telemedicine group that I trusted.

As I transition into the next phase of my career, the word retirement seems absurd considering how involved I am in the future of medicine and restoring scientific integrity to our country, and world. However, nothing caps my career quite like those emails, which I read with increasing joy and less duty today more than ever.

In so many words, I now regularly hear, "Professor Risch, your advice saved my life." To say that this has been the most satisfying moment of my career so far is an understatement. I have what I call my "baby papers," research publications where I think that I did my most clever or most important scientific contributions. Some of these have won academic or large financial prizes and I am justifiably proud of them, but they pale in personal satisfaction compared to the people whose lives I have helped. They came to me because I have had a sizable media following hundreds of media appearances—public appearances that are not all that comfortable for me. After all, my intellectual home is in the laboratory, on the computer, with study staff, doing science.

Over the last two years, however, I have taken on the role that someone with career authority must stand up for in expressing objective, truthful science. I am not willing to lie and say that Nature says something other than what it says. Either a drug works for a disease or it doesn't. My job is to "translate Nature into English" as objectively as I can, and that's what I have striven to do.

And to every person who listened and acted upon my sound, scientific findings; to all of you who refused to adopt the fear porn perpetuated in mass media; for those of you who found your voice and didn't sit back, trusting a plan with no empirical evidence; for those of you who resisted and withstood the pressure of often authentic and yet misguided friends, family members, or peers, I applaud you. I honor you. It is you who are brave. Thank you for your bravery.

I'm just a scientist trying to tell the truth as best I can.

Dr. Harvey Risch

Chapter Four Takeaways

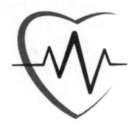

As I said in introducing Dr. Risch: science is irrefutable. You cannot read what Dr. Risch has so eloquently written and not be left with a sense of profound finality and purpose. Bad science is corrupting the way we deliver healthcare in this country.

Plausibility fraud turns theory into fact, taking the summative or opening lines of a paper and presenting that as the science, ignoring the pages of research, experiment, and study that provide insight, proof, or sometimes, the margin of error into that headline.

Science is also frequently mislabeled. Randomized trials are not necessarily that, especially when performed over small samples. Yet these trials will be presented as such, with those results used to override those of more substantial science to fit the agenda of the backer: Big Pharma, the media, and those with a stake.

The request of Dr. Risch, myself, and everyone here at TWC, is that you, as part of your own health-accountability journey, do the reading behind the studies. Arm yourself with the knowledge to challenge that which is wrong and take ownership of yourself. We are here to help you on that journey.

Also, as Dr. Risch mentions, good healthcare is more accessible than ever, if you know where to look and go to the right people. Telehealth is on the rise, and those without access to the privilege of top-end private healthcare are reaping the benefits of a system that can save the user money by avoiding unnecessary appointments. The right telehealth provider, be that us or another suitably equipped provider, can examine your issues and symptoms and make the right recommendation, irrespective of how long that takes.

We aim to always provide the most scientifically accurate information and to pass that knowledge not just to you, but to the wider medical community in a process that allows us to assist in the enlightening of the entire industry.

Foster Coulson

Dr. Richard Amerling

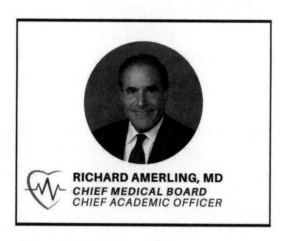

Dr. Richard Amerling is a leading authority figure on nephrology, and an active opponent of the concept of EBM, as introduced in the previous chapter. EBM, as we know, is a flawed process, and Dr. Amerling instead advocates the personalized approach of Science-Based Medicine.

Dr. Amerling has, by his sheer magnanimity, brought many people into the fold, despite his own ill-designed ostracization from a medical community that he helped to create. In early the pandemic, he worked in the Caribbean - Grenada, to be precise - and was instrumental in establishing a hitherto unseen Nephrology Program on the island. He has seen firsthand the fallacy of the investigative gene-based therapy for COVID-19 when, as the island reopened to the world, supposedly "vaccinated" people brought COVID-19 with them.

He only left the island when they announced that they were themselves off to the world, not wanting to be separated in that way from his family in the US. When he returned, he threw himself into voluntary work to help an ailing medical system.

His frontline observations and expertise have helped him identify the two greatest medical crimes of their respective centuries: the food pyramid crime of the 20th century, and the prolonged pandemic crime of the 21st century.

I won't go into any detail here, I'll let him do that, but his observations are fascinating and lay clear the exploitation of the American public by the medical institutions that are meant to serve it.

As a result of his brave defiance, I can think of no one better to train our new telehealth doctors.

Foster Coulson

Chapter 5

Conscious Medical Re-Education

"The role of the doctor is to protect patients, not to follow guidelines."
Dr. Richard Amerling

When Foster asked me to write a chapter in *The Next Wave Is Brave*, I told him that I'd been preparing content for this moment for thirty years. What you're about to read is a sobering report on the status of medicine as well as a prescription for how you and I are going to save the system through medical re-education. Along the way, we'll enjoy some rock and roll, overseas adventures, and a stunning look at how the universe conspires to synchronously prepare us for our destinies. In fact, with regard to synchronicity, my middle school years supported a critical time in my future medical career when I chose to study French as an elective course.

I was blessed to study in one of the country's most prestigious high schools, Stuyvesant, which was well-known for its science curriculum. I probably signed up for that French course because I was more interested in chasing girls than in the language, but excelling in the material gave me a favorable head start both in dating as well as my career. I studied physics at Stony Brook University after high school but was fairly distracted by, again, *les filles*, rock 'n roll, and motorcycles. This, too, will play a critical role in my professional career as a doctor.

I enjoyed physics because it gave me a sense of what real science is. One line from a priceless series The Richard Feynman Lectures on Physics has underpinned my life since that undergraduate time: "The first principle is that you must not fool yourself–and you are the easiest person to fool. So you have to be very careful about that. After you've not fooled yourself, it's easy not to fool other scientists. You just have to be honest in a conventional way after that."

I was tremendously impacted by Feynman's statement, but it didn't make physics sexier than those girls, guitars, and motorcycles. I got C's in physics in my first year, which made it impossible to raise my GPA above B+ after transferring to the City College of New York and switching to a pre-med major. Although scoring in the ninety-eighth percentile on the science part of the MCAT I couldn't get into an American medical school back then in the 1970s.

I hold no bitterness about the fact that several political agendas pushed me to the bottom of those medical school lists, including affirmative action; which was quite new at the time. Determined to become a doctor, I was accepted into medical school in Belgium at the Université Catholique de Louvain. Needless to say, that French course became quite useful.

In order to be accepted at the UCL, I was required to prepare for all of their first-year exams, *en français,* with the materials as presented by their professor. In September 1975, I passed the exams so well that I skipped their first year (a pre-med redo) and went into "real medical school" second year with only a month to prepare. *It was the proudest achievement of my life to that point.*

The Belgian curriculum was rigorous and science-based, so I was grateful for my background at Stuyvesant and in my undergrad. After clerkships in the UK in London and Edinburgh, Scotland, I graduated with honors and landed back stateside at New York Hospital, Queens (then Booth Memorial Hospital) where I did an internship, residency, and chief residency in Internal Medicine.

Like many young doctors, I was on call every two or three nights, admitting sick patients and putting out fires all night. On a good night,

I might get twenty minutes to close my eyes, then take a shower and put on a clean shirt.

I did this for three years, fueled by the Belgian approach to thinking creatively about diagnosis and treatment. With total humility, they are probably still talking about the astounding diagnoses I made to this day. After this initiation into practicing medicine, I became the Chief Resident at the hospital, but mostly I was teaching and completing administration. One of my favorite parts of the job was planning a weekly conference where we would host an expert in some area. I went out of my way to invite top-line people and well-known doctors from around the country. To this day, I love organizing conferences and positively cannot wait to recommence this work with TWC.

Synchronizing the Band

French was an accidental project that turned out to be the foundation for my entrance into medical school, as the universe would have it. I love science and was fortunate to have studied at one of the oldest medical schools in the world, known for their strong scientific curriculum, but two additional loves underpin my life and the role I now have as a general in the battle to save medical education in America: sailing and bass playing.

Playing the bass and music is a preoccupation and passion in my life. As a bass player, you have to hold the band together, uniting the rhythm section (the drums) with the harmony, and the guitars with the pianos. The bass player doesn't mind working in the background to make others look and sound good.

From the time I orchestrated care, diagnosis, and treatments in the ICU to today, I again have the opportunity to help the other superstars in this book to perform at their highest level as we work together towards a common goal. This is the role of the bass player.

Getting people to synchronize and function together as a team is also the role of the skipper of a racing sailboat. Sailboat racing, like medicine, is a challenging sport, but when you find people who work well together and you can get the most out of them, it's, well, smooth sailing–particularly when you're guided by love. I love my colleagues here at TWC, and although we're going to have to tread through some dark places, you'll see that our mission isn't to rehash the past but to create a better tomorrow.

Synchronizing the band, or getting the crew to work well together has prepared me well for working with The Wellness Company.

Zen & The Art of Health Maintenance

In another instance of my hobbies bleeding into my medical practice synchronously, I enjoyed a book in college called *Zen and the Art of Motorcycle Maintenance* by Robert M. Persig.

The protagonist's goal in the book was the search for a working definition of the word quality. Thing is, he couldn't come up with it. He sought wisdom from the Greeks, the Sophists, and other philosophers. Observing a mechanic working on his motorcycle, not thinking but interacting, Persig concludes that interaction is where the quality occurs.

Zen and The Art of Motorcycle Maintenance is a perfect analogy for medical care. The quality of medicine has to do with the patient-physician relationship. The eureka moment happened for me while listening to a colleague lecture about quality assurance in the dialysis clinic. In my observation, I realized that he was lecturing without one key control: a viable definition of quality. Persig ultimately determines that: "Quality couldn't be independently related with either the subject or the object but could be found only in the relationship of the two with each other. It is the point at which subject and object meet. Quality is not a thing. It is an event. It is the event at which the subject becomes aware of the object."

Current definitions of quality healthcare are tied to outcomes. Practices or procedures associated with good outcomes are retrospectively labeled as high quality. However, retrospective studies, which make up the bulk of medical literature, are difficult to interpret because many uncontrolled variables may have influenced the outcome. One obvious confounding variable is the underlying health of the population studied. Reports may show decent outcomes, but perhaps the preselected patient population was relatively healthy to begin with? An analogy with higher education would be if a university boasts the success of its graduates; is that due to the quality of education? Or is it because their students were handpicked from the cream of applicants who would be more likely to succeed in any setting?

The only way to conclude that a given treatment affected an outcome would be to perform a prospective randomized, double-blind, placebo-controlled study. We can conclude a treatment is effective if more patients in the treatment group respond favorably with statistical significance. However, as my distinguished colleague, Dr. Harvey Risch points out, it is very easy for a sponsor (i.e. Pharma) to manipulate these studies to produce, or give the appearance of a desired result.

I'll now introduce a concept that my colleague Dr. Harvey Risch touched upon in Chapter Four: Evidence-Based Medicine, or EBM.

EBM is a movement that started in Canada during the 1990s with the lofty goal of incorporating so-called "best evidence" into medical decision-making. Sadly, it rapidly became a pseudoscientific cult that was hijacked by Pharma to create "practice guidelines" that invariably instruct doctors to prescribe more drugs.

Physicians deal with individual patients with varying demographics, dynamics, histories, and even cultures, which play a large role in medical prognosis, treatment decisions, and adoption by the patients. EBM can, at best, provide a statistical likelihood that a patient will respond favorably to a specific treatment. However, physicians must treat patients individually, not based on statistical studies that are often flawed or biased. This requires discernment, intuition, and judgment. These come from clinical experience, something that is relegated to the lower levels of the EBM hierarchy of "evidence."

The idea that a panel of experts (most of whom have considerable financial conflicts of interest) can define "best evidence" and dictate medical practice to everyone is bizarre and unacceptable on its face. Yet, that is exactly what has occurred and has led to what I've been calling medical tyranny or medical fascism. Doctors who dare step outside the official guidelines are being accused of spreading misinformation or disinformation.

Guidelines are useless when dealing with a new problem. Persig states in *Zen*, "Technology presumes there's just one right way to do things and there never is . . . the art of the work is just as dependent upon your own mind and spirit as it is upon the material of the machine. That's why you need peace of mind." Twenty years in advance of the guidelines or EBM movement, Persig destroys the argument with this craftsman analogy:

> *"Sometime look at a novice workman or a bad workman and compare his expression with that of a craftsman whose work you know is excellent and you'll see the difference. The craftsman isn't ever following a single line of instruction. He's making decisions as he goes along. For that reason he'll be absorbed and attentive to what he's doing even though he doesn't deliberately contrive this. His motions and the machine are in a kind of harmony.* **He isn't following any set of written instructions because the nature of the material at hand determines his thoughts and motions, which simultaneously change the nature of the material at hand. The material and his thoughts are changing together in a progression of changes until his mind's at rest at the same time the material's right."** *(bold emphasis added)*

Quality in Healthcare

I first published *Zen and the Art of Health Maintenance* in 2004 because I lamented the increasing deterioration of the patient-physician relationship with every independent doctor who sold his or her practice to a larger corporate healthcare organization and every political initiative that threatened that sacred relationship. Healing occurs as a result of quality patient-physician relationships; it has nothing to do with achieving numerical targets. Your cholesterol or diabetes targets for the month have nothing to do with the patient and physician. I knew that EBM initiatives would worsen the quality of healthcare.

Quality in healthcare is predicated on the quality of the physician-patient relationship. The moment a patient feels compassion from his physician, that sparks the healing process. As Drs Peter and Harvey have excellently illustrated in this book, financial incentives (twenty percent kickbacks on the use of Remdesivir, anyone?) and threats from their hospital corporations interfere with the quality and purity of that patient-physician relationship.

The mere complication and staff requirements of Medicare and Medicaid reimbursements have distanced doctors from quality care. Instead of spending time with or thinking about their patients, physicians are burdened with extra staff, books, and computers, and must navigate a labyrinth of complex billing procedures. These burdens have collectively led to a mass exodus of physicians out of private practice and into the arms of large hospital corporations where their autonomy is constrained. In the 1980s and 90s, most doctors worked in private practice. Today, the vast majority of doctors work in a corporate system. The private independent physician was the backbone of quality medical care in a community, thought of similarly to a village elder. Throughout history, physicians have long sat at the center of the community. Today, independent, community-driven physicians are on the verge of extinction.

At TWC we are committed to the Hippocratic ideal that doctors place the interest of their patients above all else.

Dr. Vladimir Zelenko stated that had he sold his practice to a larger institution, he could never have created the life-saving Zelenko Protocol that is now attributed to saving millions of lives during the pandemic.

The Physicians' Declaration of Independence

In the late 1980s and early 90s, after I had completed about ten years of post-graduate training, I got involved with the fight against a planned takeover of the medical system by the Clintons: HillaryCare. I was an ardent foe of socialized medicine, and I knew that's where they were headed. I wrote a few letters to journals and some articles and joined the Association of American Physicians and Surgeons, a venerable organization devoted to maintaining freedom in medicine, independent medical practice, and the patient-physician relationship.

It was fascinating to learn that my colleague, Dr. Heather Gessling, was involved with a recent Physicians' Declaration of Independence related to COVID-19 policy. In 2010, I published a PDOI on the AAPS website in response to the looming ObamaCare legislation. In it, I wrote:

"When in the Course of Human Events, it becomes necessary for the members of a Profession to dissolve the Financial Arrangements which have connected them with Medicare, Medicaid, assorted Health Maintenance Organizations, and diverse Third Party Payers and to assume among the other Professions of the Earth, the separate and equal station to which the Laws of Nature and of Nature's God entitle them, a decent respect to the opinions of Mankind requires that they should declare the causes which impel them to the separation.

We hold these truths to be self-evident: that the Physician's primary responsibility is toward the Patient; that to assure the sanctity of this relationship, payment for service should be decided between Physician and Patient, and that, as in all transactions in a free society, this payment be mutually agreeable. Only such a Financial Arrangement will guarantee the highest level of Commitment and

Service of the Physician to the Patient, restrain Outside Influence on Decision-Making, and assure that personal information be kept confidential.

The Financial Arrangements between Physicians and the Third Parties have become so destructive to the Patient-Physician relationship, and to the Medical Profession as a whole, that it is the Right, and Obligation, of the Members of the Profession to abolish them. Prudence will dictate that arrangements long established should not be changed for light and transient causes; and accordingly all experience has shown, that Physicians are more disposed to suffer, while evils are sufferable, than to right themselves by abolishing the forms to which they are accustomed. But when a long train of abuses and usurpations evinces a design to reduce them under Absolute Despotism, it is their Right; it is their Duty, to throw off such arrangements, and to provide new Guards for their future security.

Such has been the patient sufferance of the members of this Profession; and such is now the necessity that constrains them to alter their former Financial Arrangements. The history of the present system is a history of repeated injuries and usurpations, all having in direct effect the establishment of an absolute Tyranny over the Medical Profession." See: https://aapsonline.org/physicians-declaration-of-independence/

It was obvious that medical practice was being undermined by third-party payment, and that the only way to restore the patient-physician relationship was for doctors to opt out of these various schemes and establish direct pay practices. This is still true and even more urgent today.

The Crime of the Century

With that sub-headline, I bet you thought I was going to dive straight into a COVID-19 manmade bioweapon story, eh? Unfortunately, something equally dark and sinister preceded this pandemic and illustrates classically how our guidelines are corrupt, and why we must return to medicine based on real science and the centrality of the patient-physician relationship.

Around the late 1970s and then revised again in 1980, came Dietary Guidelines for Americans. The DGA directs people to avoid saturated (animal) fat and to consume half their calories from carbohydrates ("the food pyramid.") It's almost unthinkable. This is a formula for obesity. When I grew up in the 1950s, 60s, and 70s, there were very few obese people. Now the sad fact is that the majority of the population is overweight and slim people stand out.

Behind the DGA was an effort to sell cheap, industrially produced vegetable seed oils like Crisco from companies such as Proctor and Gamble. Ancel Keys, a so-called physiologist, was obsessed with the idea that dietary saturated fat caused coronary artery disease by increasing cholesterol levels. This became known as the "Diet-Heart Hypothesis." He conducted two population studies looking to correlate dietary fat intake with rates of heart disease. Both showed what appeared to be a linear relationship between the two, but it became obvious that he cherry-picked the countries to support his hypothesis, conveniently omitting France, for example.

The French consume enormous amounts of fat yet remain slim and relatively free of heart disease. Keys was hired by the American Heart Association (AHA) which helped his ideas to become dominant. The AHA received a $1.6 million grant from P&G and relentlessly pushed the low-fat concept, which continues to this day.

The DGA harmed millions of people and dramatically demonstrated the risk of central health policy. Obesity, which is a marker for serious metabolic disease, followed the adoption of low-fat, high-carb recommendations.

This isn't intended to shame anybody. I believe that the public was misdirected - even criminally so - to follow guidelines that lined corporate pockets with money and collective waistlines with fat. Today, obesity has become normalized, and calling out a clearly unhealthy body is labeled as fat shaming. The amount of harm caused by these dietary guidelines and the incorporation of vegetable oils into the American diet is incalculable.

The other major consequence of the DGA was the addition by the food industry of massive amounts of sugar (later, high fructose corn syrup) into virtually all processed food. Fructose, which is 50-55 percent of sugar (sucrose) is obligatorily metabolized to triglycerides (fat) in the liver and is a primary cause of fatty liver, insulin resistance, and metabolic syndrome.

We have forty years of misinformation to debunk and redirect people towards true health and wellness. The Wellness Company seeks to re-educate doctors and the public that have been deceived by the food industry into eating toxic "foods" and by the pharmaceutical industry who pocket billions by "treating" the resulting diseases.

My Exit from Corporate Medicine

Armed with a growing resentment of medical care, the exodus of doctors from independent practices, the aggressive domination of insurance companies and hospital corporations in patient-physician relationships and the subsequent degradation of Quality Care, I left my practice in 2016. As with all Amerling stories, this one too is full of breathtaking synchronicity.

From 1990 to 2016 I worked as a staff nephrologist in New York at Beth Israel Medical Center–a large academically-oriented hospital that served Manhattan's Lower East Side and East Village.

BI was a wonderful community staffed by excellent clinicians, both private and full-time, that I interacted with daily. We provided fantastic care and were free to practice the kind of medicine that we felt was best. It was, even then, a dying breed and a breath of fresh air. It was a major teaching hospital with a large house staff of interns, residents, and fellows in training. We had a fellowship program in Nephrology and produced a long string of excellent nephrologists.

Though I was mostly involved with clinical work and had no "protected time," I was able to conduct some clinical research and presented regularly at major conferences. At several of these, I would run into Dr. Peter McCullough, whose interests in heart-kidney interactions (cardiorenal syndrome) intersected with mine.

We became friends over fifteen years ago. If you had told me way back then that we would be fighting together to preserve medical freedom, that Peter would be leading the fight, and that we would be standing shoulder-to-shoulder in this battle, I would have thought you were stark-raving mad. Another friend and former colleague from those halcyon days is Dr. Pierre Kory, who ran the ICU at BI for several years. Like Peter, Pierre became an accidental hero by simply standing up for patients and acting like all doctors should have acted in the face of a devastating new disease.

In 2014, the hospital was taken over by Mount Sinai. Although the acquisition was sold as a partnership, it was, in effect, a hostile takeover. Mount Sinai in New York had a long and glorious history as a top teaching hospital and medical school, but by that time had "gone corporate," leading to a catastrophic decline in quality.

It was during this time that I began to see elements of the perversion discussed in previous chapters of this book. People were treated by numbers and as numbers. Virtually all the division chiefs and experienced doctors were either fired or demoted. These caring and competent clinicians were deemed too expensive. We were concerned with quantity over Quality. I was dumbfounded when younger, more inexperienced, and essentially unqualified doctors replaced older, more suitably qualified ones.

At the time, I held the academic rank of Associate Professor but knew I wouldn't be advanced. The President of Mount Sinai was a psychiatrist by the name of Ken Davis who had written a self-serving op-ed piece for the *Wall Street Journal* extolling the benefits of hospital mergers and treatment based on "population health." Seething, I sent a response indicating that there was not enough information in population studies to make clinical decisions and that treatments based on "population health" harm individual patients. Letter writing, by the way, is another of my hobbies. Over the years I've had over fifty letters to the editor published by the *New York Times, The Wall Street Journal,* and others.

That letter probably sealed my fate with Mount Sinai, but I wasn't looking for a long-term relationship anyway. By that time, I'd been receiving calls from the new Division Chief saying that my electronic health records had to be signed. They weren't pressuring me to sign off my charts because I was absent-minded or disorganized. Rather, because everything was digital, unless my charts were signed off on, they couldn't bill. Nobody recognized the quality of my care but assertively urged me to sign off on my charts so that they could get paid.

The practice environment deteriorated over the following two years; the writing was clearly on the wall.

Finally, on a cold morning in January, I committed in my heart that I would get out. That exact day I was riding the subway on the East Side from my apartment to audition for a friend's church music ensemble. On the journey, I noticed an advertisement for St. George's University in Grenada, a series of buildings that resembled a luxury hotel resort with white stucco buildings and salmon-colored roofs sitting at the edge of True Blue Bay in the Caribbean Sea. The rancid taste in my mouth from the last two years vanished and I could practically taste the salty sea air and visualize myself sailing in the turquoise waters. Needless to say, the universe didn't have to twist my arm too much.

I applied for an Associate Professor level position in the Department of Clinical Skills. As a classically trained and highly experienced clinician, this was a job I could do with one hand tied behind my back. After a few interviews in Grenada, I returned to New York and closed my practice at Beth Israel/Sinai to start my new career at the level of full professor in Grenada (based on my semi-impressive curriculum vitae and double board certification, I was promoted to full professor). My daughter was finishing college at the time and my son was finishing boarding school on his way to college, so the timing was pretty near perfect in my life. As you can see, this is a running theme in my life's story.

I look back on my time in Grenada as a wonderful adventure, a truly once-in-a-lifetime experience. I picked up a racing sailboat and sailed in those electric blue and turquoise waters as often as possible. I played bass with excellent musicians almost every week at the local brewery, but more importantly, I found joy in teaching medicine to the next generation of doctors.

A New Vision for The Future of Medicine

Ever since the 1980s, I noticed something fishy in the way we were conducting medicine, educating the public, and, most importantly, educating our doctors. Medicine was falling off the rails. I relished the opportunity to illuminate the art of medicine, quality of care, and to warn my students about the dangers of Evidence-Based Medicine. What surprised me with these young MD hopefuls was the ratio of education they were getting in basic sciences versus oddly unscientific education.

A good medical history is arguably the crux of clinical diagnosis, and a vital skill for every physician to acquire. I was mildly shocked to discover they were being taught only the history form, without the essential purpose or technique that allowed for the attainment of a differential diagnosis.

Then, students were taught to work through a list of standard questions that rarely helped, and that were open-ended rather than focused. They never failed to take a sexual history, even when it had nothing to do with the patient's complaint. They always asked if vaccinations were up to date: *always*. These students, who were grossly lacking in knowledge of basic sciences, were now directed to take a version of a medical history that was frankly worthless. They were doing little more than filling in a template–something the secretary in the front office could do just as easily.

In order to take a meaningful medical history, it's important to ask very specific, not generic, questions. For instance, you can figure out by asking focused questions whether chest pain is likely due to a heart attack, muscular problem, or an esophageal spasm. And for God's sake, don't waste time asking about vaccination and sexual history when somebody is experiencing chest pain. I'd almost be laughing reading that sentence again if the implications weren't so mortal.

One day, I happened to read through a Pharmacology lecture on diabetes that was little more than a recitation of all the different classes of diabetes medications. I emailed the professor and asked if he was aware that a high-fat, low-carb diet could reverse Type 2 Diabetes. He never responded.

For the love of God, I thought, are they learning to medicate people, or to heal them? What does it mean to be a doctor anymore? Are we training puppets with Big Pharma pulling the strings? Are they learning to treat numbers or human beings? Are there any doctors coming out of medical school today who understand quality care? Are we merely soldiers for Big Pharma agendas? Do these kids who get the honor of an MD title have measurably more skill than the guy who pressed buttons on the espresso machine this morning at my local coffee shop? What makes us special? What makes us valuable? What makes us healers? Or, are we intentionally not being trained to heal?

I spoke with the Dean of Basic Science; a man I considered a friend and somebody I respected. He had achieved and published a lot, and was creative in his field of anatomy–which is impressive given that anatomy doesn't change all that much. He cleverly suggested that I create an elective course contrasting the Evidence-Based Medicine approach with a Science-Based approach. Shortly thereafter, I proposed a course to the curriculum committee. I called it *Medicine by First Principles,* inspired by an interview during which Elon Musk described how he approached problem-solving. Musk said that when confronted with a problem, go back to what you absolutely know to be true.

In medicine, the first principles are the basic sciences and the clinical presentation of a disease. Take my Type 2 Diabetes example: the EBM approach hammers the patients with drugs and insulin to reduce blood sugar. This causes weight gain and worsens their underlying metabolic syndrome. Type 2 Diabetes is a late manifestation of metabolic syndrome; high blood sugar is merely a symptom. When you reduce sugar and carb intake and get rid of vegetable oils, you can reverse Type 2 Diabetes. It's really not that difficult and I've done it many times.

As a nephrologist, hypertension is in my realm of expertise. The entire notion of "essential hypertension" is, in my view, bogus. In most cases, we do know what is causing hypertension. Rather than looking at a patient simplistically, when you approach hypertension with an understanding of pathophysiology you can establish more effective treatments and often reverse it.

The Pharma model perpetuates the concept that we have this chronic disease and are destined to take pills for life. It's a solid business plan, especially when you change blood pressure targets with the purpose of increasing your revenue. Lowering blood pressure targets through bought-and-paid-for guideline panels is an effective way to get millions more people stuck in a drug treatment model.

To the readers of this book, my opinions probably sound pretty sane, humane, and even urgent. Nevertheless, *Medicine by First Principles* was not approved, not even as an elective course.

One of my duties in Grenada was to see patients at the General Hospital, which was a state-run hospital based out of an old military barrack up a hill. We used to say that if you could get to the hospital up that hill, you probably didn't have a real heart attack. In just the short time I worked there I lamented seeing a handful of well-trained doctors pushed out in favor of doctors for hire - mostly from Cuba - of "variable quality." Most of these doctors had a great deal of trouble with the English language, and the hospital care by American standards was atrocious. I witnessed firsthand some horrific outcomes in patients who died unnecessarily as a result of the care that they received. I tried to start a dialysis program in the hospital based on Peritoneal Dialysis, but that was an uphill battle, to say the least.

I was successful in accomplishing diabetes reversal in many patients, and my students learned a lot through the process of seeing me deliver quality care. I purchased a handheld ultrasound device with my own money and began conducting an ultrasound clinic that would allow me to visualize the kidneys or bladder. I was able to perform relatively decent echocardiograms on patients in the clinic.

The island of Grenada is made more beautiful by the most wonderful, friendly people in the world. Among my fondest memories is rowing a custom-built twelve-foot dinghy in the bay. My little house overlooked the bay and the ocean, and I loved to grill meat on the patio and watch for the proverbial green flash. My phone grew full of sunset pictures.

Although I was acutely aware of the degradation of medicine around me, I lived a simple life. I miss the constant companionship of Simba, a wonderful part Golden Retriever, part Belgian Malinois dog whose owner allowed him to roam the neighborhood. She tells me that around sunset, he often hangs around in front of the door to my old home and cries. When I think of that home, that view, and that sweet dog I remember that although it was too short a time, I was guided by some compassionate and loving force to influence students as well as make a few friends along the way.

One friend I'll never forget was a doctor who was struggling with kidney failure while we worked together on the dialysis program. She wasn't doing well, and I personally intervened several times at critical moments in the course of her illness to save her life with emergency dialysis treatments. I could see that without a kidney transplant, her days were numbered. Thankfully, we were in touch with a group of volunteer doctors who had come down to the island to help with our program's surgical procedures. Through this contact, we were able to arrange for a kidney transplant to be performed in Guyana, with her son as the donor. It took about a year to arrange the paperwork, raise funds, and get everything lined up. The surgery was technically challenging and it took three months for kidney function to kick in, but kick in it did, and it's still going strong. This was one of the most satisfying clinical experiences of my career. I had already left Grenada to volunteer in New York's Bellevue Hospital in the spring of 2020 and did not get to see my friend and colleague transformed to good health thanks to some wonderful surgeons, her amazing son, and God. I remain an unofficial consultant on the Nephrology Program that I started and that she now runs. Using telemedicine, I still consult with some of my patients in Grenada despite the fact that I have been gone now for well over two years.

They Were Not Gonna Let It End

I want to highlight the series of events that led me to leave Grenada as they will inform the work I'm doing today to help restore exceptional medical education after at least forty years of care, compassion, and common sense being aggressively replaced with EBM and Big Pharma corruption.

In early 2020, I thought COVID-19 was the subject of media fascination and a degree of overhype. I was experiencing the common ex-pat symptom of looking at the rest of the world like they were too urgent, too hurried, and they needed a week or two on island time to calm down and reset. To my chagrin, the University closed and most of the students were sent home, with just a few hundred remaining on the island. They immediately switched to online teaching and exams. I lingered on the island until the government declared that they were going to close the airport and isolate the island from the rest of the world. That was the straw that broke the camel's back—my children were in the States and I couldn't fathom being away from them for some indefinite period. I left all my things on the island and flew back to the States at the end of March, assuming I'd be going back in a few months.

Seeing that New York City was being hit hard - mostly among nursing home patients - I added my name to a burgeoning list of volunteers. An old colleague at the Manhattan VA emailed me and reported that they were seeing a lot of kidney failure and with a doctor ill and out of commission due to COVID-19, they were struggling and he invited me to come. I volunteered at Bellevue and Manhattan VA, rounding with their doctors and assisting with their dialysis program. In a few weeks, they put together a very good acute peritoneal dialysis program. We were flying by the seat of our pants without randomized trials for anything. It was terrifying; we knew very little about how to treat the most sick patients. On the other hand, it was invigorating to see medicine advance in real-time based on experience and knowledge of medicine and pathophysiology. Sadly, we lost a lot of patients. The most painful part of that experience was watching patients die alone in the ICU without their families.

After a month, the ICU was no longer busy and I thought, to all intents and purposes, that the pandemic was over. However, it soon became clear they were not going to let it end. I see now that this was a way to destroy the economy, the Trump presidency, and a way to keep people living in fear. Fear is where they are most easy to control and manipulate.

A moment of awakening for me was when the virus was clearly over but the fear continued with massive testing of asymptomatic individuals with a high cycle PCR test that was creating waves of false positives.

The lockdowns were horrific. The masking was horrific. Lives were being destroyed over a pandemic that had already ended. If the food pyramid was the crime of the 20th Century, this was the crime of the 21st Century. In August, I eagerly wanted to return to Grenada but the island was still closed, subject to the imposition of a rigid quarantine and curfew; I wasn't going to return to a police state.

I reoccupied my NYC apartment, continued teaching online, and continued helping my patients in Grenada through telemedicine. The threat of a vaccine mandate at SGU terrified me, and I anticipated that my refusal to comply would eventually see me canceled. In January 2021, I sold my apartment in New York and prepared to get back to the University and the clinic.

A Failure of Courage

In late January 2021, I did return to the clinic in Grenada and was encouraged by the anti-vaccine stance of the Chief of the Clinical Skills Division. However, in April the University issued a vaccine mandate for all staff, faculty, and students. Sadly, he caved and complied when his job was threatened; it's worth noting how many people didn't want the shot but were not brave enough to stand their ground and think themselves out of a menacing situation.

Grenadians are smart people; ninety percent of them didn't want the COVID-19 investigational gene-based therapy commonly called a "vaccine." Grenada experienced a mild COVID-19 outbreak in 2020 with only eight hospitalizations and no deaths due to my colleagues' wise use of hydroxychloroquine. They had zero cases for over a year. Although the government pushed vaccination, only about thirty percent of the population complied. When their quarantine requirement was relaxed for travelers with a vax card, those vaccinated visitors brought with them a massive outbreak of what we believe was the Delta variant, resulting in over two hundred deaths.

Among those who had been adamantly against the "vaccine" were most of the people working in my division when I returned to the island in January 2021. Secretaries, patients, and even the tech department were adamantly opposed to the shot. The most tragic part of my colleague's failure of courage was that his decision to comply trickled down to the rest of the division; they were then given an impossible choice: comply or lose their job. Had this colleague been brave, these souls would have been spared the anguish of having to accept a medical procedure they simply did not want. We were important enough to the school that had we united and resisted, we would have won. I resisted and was summarily placed on administrative leave without pay, returning to the States in July 2021 and officially terminated in January 2022. My response is worth a look:

On Fri, Jul 16, 2021 at 11:18 AM Richard Amerling <RAmerlin@ sgu.edu> wrote:

Dear Dr. Olds,

Thanks again for taking the time to discuss the Covid vaccine issue with me.

The debate over a vaccine mandate at SGU comes down to dissonance between individual and public health decision-making. Since public health measures can be used to impose a collectivist tyranny (see eugenics), and SGU is primarily a School of Medicine, we should come down on the side of Hippocratic medical ethics, putting our patients' benefit first and doing no harm. The vast majority of students, for example, have near-zero risk of mortality (and serious morbidity) from Covid. For them, risk vs benefit analysis argues against taking an investigational product with no long-term safety data (and some alarming short-term safety issues, including almost 10,000 deaths in VAERS), since they will be highly unlikely to benefit.

Regarding public health, you said that with local community spread there could be over a thousand dead in Grenada! This is a shocking number, but assumes a high infection fatality rate. A more reasonable estimated IFR of 0.15% based on a John P Ioannidis meta-analysis (https://pubmed.ncbi.nlm.nih.gov/33768536/) gives a worst-case scenario of 100 deaths. This number assumes the entire population of 100k is infected, and no access to early treatment. The initial experience with Covid in Grenada, when the virus was new and still highly virulent, produced only a handful of hospitalizations. All of these recovered with hydroxychloroquine and supplemental oxygen. Our esteemed colleague Dr. Dolland Noel heroically took care of these patients. Based on his experience, and that of many others, early treatment with hydroxychloroquine is effective (you can add to that ivermectin.)

Could the Grenada General Hospital be overwhelmed? The truth is they are overwhelmed on a daily basis and can barely treat many basic diseases. Grenadians die there every day from acute coronary syndromes, heart failure, kidney failure, complications of diabetes, cirrhosis, etc. I've seen more amputations in a few years than in my entire career in NYC. Mechanical ventilation carried a >70% mortality in the early cohorts hospitalized in NYC and elsewhere. There are ventilators at the GGH, but if a Covid patient requires one, they are very likely not going to survive.

My skepticism about the Covid vaccine is based on a variety of factors:

1) >30 years' experience as a scientifically trained nephrologist, with intimate knowledge of how Pharma influences and corrupts medical education and practice.

2) Frontline experience with the first wave of Covid patients hospitalized at Bellevue and the Manhattan VA last spring and summer

3) Closely following the medical literature, and reports from reputable physicians actually treating sick patients. Many of these

intrepid doctors are being censored and harassed, which makes the truth of their messages more compelling. The demonization of HCQ (see the fake Lancet study, for example, retracted after 10 days), and more recently ivermectin, is not based in fact or science. While we can debate the efficacy of these agents, they are certainly not dangerous. This campaign smacks of a Big Pharma op, and can be seen as intended to create and maintain the demand for the vaccines, and for the Emergency Use Authorization.

4) After the initial wave subsided last summer, life should have returned to normal. But the fear-mongering media, government officials, the CDC, and WHO pushed the "casedemic," based on over-amplified PCR tests done inappropriately in tens of millions of asymptomatic individuals. Many if not most of these asymptomatic "cases" were false positives. And since when in medicine do we define a "case" based on a single lab test, and a controversial one at that?

5) The unprecedented push, worldwide, to vaccinate every single human being regardless of underlying health status, risk of Covid mortality, age, pregnancy, prior immunity, etc., through advertising, bribes, and outright coercion, is extremely troubling in and of itself. It is quite simply unjustified for a virus that the vast majority of the population brush off with mild or no symptoms. The current strains, including Delta, are much less virulent than the original. This is the natural history of viral epidemics—Indolent strains have a survival advantage.

6) Selling the shots based on impressive relative risk reduction, while downplaying the adverse events is right out of the Pfizer/ Pharma playbook. The actual risk reduction with the Pfizer product is 0.7%, and barely over 1% for Moderna. They don't stop transmission, as evidenced by large numbers of so-called breakthrough cases. Recall the Tamiflu scandal: After the source

data was pulled out of the sponsor by a 3-year-long legal battle, the drug was shown to be no more effective than placebo, and with some serious downsides!

7) The spike protein, produced by the mRNA and DNA-based products, is pathogenic, and widely disseminated throughout the body.

8) The official narrative and recommendations, backed by most of the media, the CDC, the WHO, Fauci, etc have been wildly inconsistent and mostly wrong, starting with the absurd Neil Ferguson models out of the Imperial College of London (heavily financed by Gates, China, by the way). Covid-19 was produced in the lab by Ralph Baric of UNC and Zheng-Li Shi of the Wuhan Institute of Virology, funded partially by Tony Fauci's NIAID. Lockdowns, masks, distancing, have not decreased viral spread, but have caused enormous harm (especially lockdowns). Closing schools and masking kids are particularly grievous errors. The virus poses serious risks for the very elderly, and those with metabolic syndrome. Quarantining the healthy, low-risk population never made sense. Asymptomatic transmission is virtually non-existent. Previous infection produces durable, broad immunity.

None of the current vaccines has completed Phase 3 trials so there is no long-term data on efficacy or safety and therefore none are FDA approved. They are still experimental. I have no issue with encouraging staff and students to get these shots, particularly those at high risk, but coercion based on loss of salary or denial of in-person education is a bridge too far. We cross it at our peril.

SGU will be morally, if not legally, liable for severe adverse events related to a coerced vaccination. This could be ruinous, and with thousands of staff and students it's naïve to think we will be spared.

Having been "on the ground" in Grenada for four of the last six months, I can tell you with certainty the vast majority of Grenadians oppose this mandate. Everyone I spoke with was strongly against it. The SGU vaccine mandate is generating considerable ill will.

Current screening at the border has been onerous but effective. PCR pre and post-travel, then after 48 hours of quarantine, is more than adequate. The vaccine mandate cannot possibly improve over zero Covid. It is all risk for no benefit. Any "cases" that slip through are very likely to be mild, and can be treated effectively with HCQ and IVM. The initial surge last spring was fearsome; what we face now is not.

I strongly oppose the Covid vaccine mandate on medical, scientific, moral and ethical grounds. I'm disappointed, but not surprised, that Nicky Steele (perhaps following SGU) is imposing a vaccine mandate for non-resident travelers to Grenada. This will add zero benefit but further injure the local economy.

As for myself, a healthy 70-year-old in pretty decent shape, the risk of an adverse event outweighs the tiny benefit provided by the current EUA products. I survived the first wave working in the ICU providing dialysis at Bellevue; I'm not particularly worried personally about Delta or Lambda. Ivermectin and HCQ are effective, should I come down with something. Pierre Kory has been publishing and lecturing about IVM (heavily censored) for many months. We worked together for years at Beth Israel in NY; he is completely trustworthy and without conflict of interest, unlike most of the other stakeholders. He is also an SGU graduate!

Speaking of experts, Dr. Peter McCullough is a world-renowned cardiologist who has published and lectured on Covid early treatment, and on Covid in general. He is also a trusted colleague, as we know each other from the cardio-renal world, where we have both lectured. After a telemedicine consultation, Dr. McCullough filled out and signed my SGU medical exemption form. Dr. Olds, can you tell on what medical/scientific grounds it was rejected? I'm sure he would be happy to discuss with you, if you would give him a call (xxx-xxx-xxxx).

For the time being, since we are continuing online teaching for the 50% or so of students unable to return, I would be happy to participate. I am eager to return to Grenada, which has truly become my home (I sold my NYC apartment in January). I have friends, CKD/ESRD patients, a rented apartment, a few electric basses, a J24 sailboat, and a dog awaiting my return. In addition to the Renal Clinic and Dialysis Program, we are setting up a transplant program with colleagues in Guyana.

Things change, and I'm hopeful that with time and experience, both SGU and Grenada will drop their vaccine mandates. And the vaccine landscape is changing. Currently the Russian and Chinese vaccines, while almost certainly less "effective," are very likely safer as they do not involve production of spike protein. And Novavax, using a modified spike protein, looks promising. If I'm skeptical of US Pharma products, I'm doubly so about Chinese or Russian offerings. Time will tell.

Finally, you are cherished friends and colleagues. I have only the greatest respect and admiration for you. At this point in my life, my major concerns are for my kids, the future of the US, the people of Grenada, and the future of SGU. The massive global overreaction to what is a very manageable disease has done great harm. It truly grieves me that SGU and Grenada are following this destructive path.

My highest regards,

Richard Amerling, MD

PS: As this is not a scientific treatise, I did not want to clutter it with references. I can provide them for every point. If your main sources of Covid information are the mainstream media, CDC, WHO, you are not getting a full picture. Attached is a spreadsheet with links to articles and videos on Covid that you very likely have missed.

Here is my response to Vice Chancellor Dr. Rich Liebowitz after receiving the termination letter.

Dear Rich,

I take issue with the weasel language in your letter (attached): "we accept your decision that you no longer wish to fulfill the terms of your employment." As you can see below, I was quite willing to continue to teach at SGU. It was you, and the MOH, that made it impossible for me to remain physically in Grenada. SGU summarily dismissed my medical exemption request, filled out by a world leader in COVID-19. In July, I came down with symptomatic Covid that was diagnosed by a top physician and documented with acute and chronic antibodies. I am unvaccinated and truly fully immune.

Online teaching continued. You clearly did not want me around. And now, quite frankly, the feeling is mutual. I am sickened by what your mandate has done to the people of Grenada, and to SGU.

I specifically warned you in a prior email that you could not improve on zero Covid, and that countries with vaccine rollouts were experiencing major spikes in cases (Seychelles, Gibraltar, UK, Israel), hospitalizations and deaths. You ushered in double-vaccinated Delta super spreaders. Your policy brought death and destruction. You broke faith with Hippocratic Medicine, and with your many Grenadian staff, the majority of whom were strongly opposed to the shots. You forced students with sincere religious objections to take the shot or be dismissed. This is absolutely horrific, tyrannical policy.

And there was zero justification scientifically. The shots never prevented transmission, death or hospitalization. They barely worked to "reduce symptoms." The pharma-sponsored pivotal trials were pathetic. The vaccine mandates have failed miserably everywhere. They have allowed nasty variants to emerge.

SGU has destroyed its reputation as a School of Medicine. I suggest you rename it the School of Public Health and Diversity.

Richard Amerling, MD

This is the response from the President of SGU:

I think the saddest thing is to see a well-trained physician get caught up in these conspiracy theories. Our vaccine mandate didn't bring COVID to Grenada, the fact that it takes 3-5 days for infected people to test positive and poor adherence to mask and social distancing rules did. We should be proud that no fully immunized SGU faculty, staff or student died or even got very sick.

And my response to him:

> It's a conspiracy fact; a pharma op from the beginning. Why were eminent physicians speaking and writing about their success with early outpatient treatment censored? Did you approve of this?
>
> What's sad is that an eminent professor can't admit he was wrong. It was the erroneous belief, pushed by you and others, that two magic jabs actually provide immunity. This led to the relaxation of what had been an effective quarantine policy, only for the vaccinated. Once Delta got in, it was going to spread, regardless of the worthless masks and distancing.
>
> If what you say is true, and I have no way of knowing, then you dodged a major bullet. Thank God. But many others died.
>
> Even if the shots worked as advertised (and they don't) the mandate was ill-advised. It was morally wrong to force people to choose between a jab with unknown long-term effects, and their jobs.
>
> As I said in the earlier email, I consider you all friends and colleagues. I hope you understand that I had to speak my mind. And I certainly don't expect you to agree.
>
> Richard Amerling, MD

And that, my friends, is how you have a triumph of courage versus a failure. When the next wave of whatever Fauci, the CDC, the WHO, the WEF, or whoever is pulling the strings comes down the pipeline, I expect that you will be prepared. If you can't squirrel away money in preparation to lose a job because of criminally forced mandates, how can you align with people in your community in a barter economy? I loved to hear of a friend living in a rural community who aligned with a group of fellow awakened community members on Telegram where they meet regularly and keep in contact daily, committing to preparing for the next wave, because if we're united, the next wave can be truly brave.

The COVID-19 (Lack of) Response and the Tyranny of Evidence-Based Medicine

In this chapter, we have discussed the tyranny of Evidence-Based Medicine that I witnessed emerge during my forty-year career in medicine. You have likely read my story and others in this book so far and wondered why the vast majority of physicians did almost nothing to help patients in the early phases of COVID-19.

First and foremost, many physicians worldwide depend on guidelines from the World Health Organization. Rather than hopping on Telegram groups or chats with other doctors who were generating success in early treatment, many doctors twiddled their thumbs to the mortal detriment of the patients that depended on them, because the World Health Organization didn't support the use of any early treatment procedures or drugs such as Ivermectin or Hydroxychloroquine.

However, those guidelines are consistently wrong. The World Health Organization, which receives more than fifty percent of its funding from the pharmaceutical industry and the Gates Foundation, along with the CDC and FDA, are plainly corrupted. As you saw in my example with the Grenadians, it wasn't until vaccinated visitors entered the country that we had two hundred unnecessary deaths. With early treatment and the use of hydroxychloroquine, we had zero deaths over the span of an entire year.

Because most doctors have become dependent on guidelines, they have lost their ability to think critically, problem-solve, and practice real clinical medicine. When the first wave of COVID-19 hit in March and April of 2020, only the acutely ill patient was given attention. A handful of brave doctors, including Zev Zelenko in New York and Didier Raoult in Marseille, France, repurposed existing drugs such as hydroxychloroquine in early outpatient treatment. Instead of being embraced and emulated, they were censored and harassed: "These treatments are not evidence-based! Where are the randomized controlled trials?"

What we witnessed in the COVID-19 pandemic illustrated what I call the Tyranny of Evidence-Based Medicine. In this chapter, you have seen multiple examples of how EBM has deteriorated common sense and compassionate critical care to the detriment of the patient.

In their excellent book, *Tarnished Gold: The Sickness of Evidence-Based Medicine*, Steve Hickey and Hillary Roberts write:

> *"EBM encourages totalitarian medicine. It is displacing the doctor-patient unit as the ultimate decision-making authority. Peer review is used as censorship. EBM is a self-referential closed system, where critical appraisal means checking whether a study conforms to its rules. So-called evidence-based medicine wrongly claims the authority of medical and scientific gold-standards. EBM repackages and uses concepts from legal proof, in an attempt to impose a medical dictatorship."*

Doctors are immune from liability, even in the case of COVID-19, during which hundreds of thousands of souls were prematurely laid to rest, often without loved ones by their sides. Thanks to the tyranny of EBM, all those doctors have to say is, "I was just following the guidelines."

"I was just following orders" is more like it. They failed to approach COVID-19 with intelligence, science, originality, and individual care. They are guilty of grievous malpractice, they have destroyed their brand and credibility, and they have created a vacuum. The Wellness Company is stepping into that vacuum.

We're going to fill this void that was created by the abdication of the vast majority of practicing doctors.

Pushing Back Against Tyranny

When doctors are bravely committed to protecting patients and obligated by their ethics to protect them from harm, they will not comply with EBM tyranny. It is the duty of doctors to shield patients from any entity - including government programs - that put the patient in harm's way.

Doctors, because they gave up their independent status over the years and became salaried employees, gave up their profession. They became tradesmen, and poor tradesmen to boot. Had the medical profession and its leadership stood up and said, "These gene therapy shots are experimental. They do not prevent infection. They do not prevent mortality. They do not prevent hospitalization. They have the potential to cause harm. We will not comply," so much pain and unnecessary death could have been avoided, and the credibility of the medical profession could have been protected.

However, they *did* comply with what Dr. McCullough calls the "needle in every arm program." The one-size-fits-all approach to medicine perpetuated by EBM is the tyranny that I've been fighting all these years. It's what drove me to Grenada and then home again.

My profession has been hijacked by Pharma. Doctors have stopped thinking for themselves. In many ways, they have turned over their brain to the so-called expert panels to make decisions for them and their patients. If they had stayed independent, they might not have become slaves to EBM guidelines or, dare I say it, Big Pharma sell-outs. They lost their souls.

At The Wellness Company, we believe that each person is a unique individual and requires an individualized approach. We're training our telemedicine colleagues to strengthen the patient-physician relationship, to think for themselves, and to treat each patient as a unique individual with a unique problem.

We are here to be the home for the doctors who have come to their senses and are rejecting EBM, choosing instead to embrace Medicine by First Principles by using science, not evidence. Science is a process, evidence is just something we use in that scientific process. In our process of deprescribing, we want to get people off prescription drugs as much as possible.

When Dr. Simone Gold created America's Frontline Doctors (AFLDS), she set a precedent for people like our team here at TWC. She was unafraid; she created an organization that became powerful and ubiquitous in the consciousness of awakened men and women nationwide, and even across the world. When I returned home from Grenada for the second time in July 2021, I emailed Dr. Gold and asked her if I could contribute to her organization.

Acquiescing to my request, Dr. Gold asked me to research the background on the "vaccine" and conflicts of interest among the FDA vaccine committee panelists, and what I found shook me to the core. I became the Associate Medical Director at AFLDS for a period until Dr. Heather Gessling and I realized that our next mission had to be telemedicine. In essence, that's where The Wellness Company started. I was so impressed by Foster and his brave declaration that together we could change the future of medicine.

This story is a story of synchronicities starting from my middle school French class to my love of sailing and an advertisement I happened to catch on a subway train in New York one January morning. It took an act of God to help me exit my practice in New York, another to bring me to Grenada, and yet another to bring me to AFLDS where I met Dr. Heather Gessling. Collaborating with my old friend and colleague of twenty years Dr. Peter McCullough puts even further into perspective the Divine Timing, Divine Purpose, and Divine Future ahead of us all. Dr. Harvey Risch and I are kindred spirits in our criticism of the Evidence-Based Medicine approach and we are currently collaborating on a paper. I'll finally be teaching Medicine By First Principles, taking the lead in educating our telemedicine doctors. I dream of building our own medical school someday soon.

Among the mounting evidence that God exists and is good is the fact that He has led us from a dire situation to come together in this venture.

Not just Foster, our team at The Wellness Company, the doctors, and myself, but you, too.

Dr. Richard Amerling

Chapter Five Takeaways

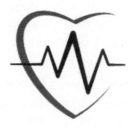

Tyranny. I agree with Dr. Amerling in that no word better describes what our broken medical system has done to the American public.

It has held them hostage by promoting unhealthy practices and forcing us to pay for the resulting treatment. Lies and misinformation about the food pyramid that caused record obesity in the 20th Century preceded a "needle in every arm" heist in the 21st.

These scandals have resulted in billions of dollars being pumped into the Biopharmaceutical Complex through a combination of private spending and taxpayer contribution. The healthcare community has, by and large, allowed itself to be duped into believing the lies, which in turn has led to the hoodwinking of the American public.

You may ask how they found this so easy. The truth is, they were already primed. EBM softened the underbelly of the physician community, taking away the necessity for individual patient care in favor of practices that relied on summaries and probabilities, not science. Once the necessity for individual study was taken away, the medical community was primed to believe whatever it was told.

Thank God then for people like Dr. Amerling and our colleagues here at The Wellness Company who did not cave to consensus. Instead, they continued to practice proper care, and so rejected the fallacy of EBM and that which it led to, outright as the farce that it is. They have not been blinded into inaction, and as a result, are perfectly primed to lead the evolution of proper healthcare in America, and hopefully, the world.

Proper healthcare is easily accessible and available to everyone at their convenience. Illness does not take days off. It does not sleep after 5 p.m. and it does not take the weekends off. It strikes when it wants, and those that are afflicted need a service that is both affordable and there for them when they need it.

That is what Dr. Amerling is going to help us create here at TWC. He will lead the frontline, training those doctors alongside his colleagues who will be there to serve you when you need it most. And he will do so because he knows, as the rest of us do, that the only way to overthrow medical tyranny is a 1776-style revolution—a revolution from the bottom-up that undermines the bottom line of the Biopharmaceutical Complex.

Foster Coulson

Dr. Jana Schmidt

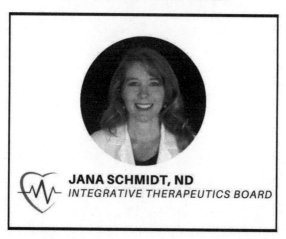

JANA SCHMIDT, ND
INTEGRATIVE THERAPEUTICS BOARD

Did you know that the vast majority of our modern medicine can trace its roots back to nature? Naturopaths, like Dr. Jana Schmidt and her Native American ancestors, have paved the way for countless advancements in modern medicine.

Why am I telling you this? I am telling you because following the advice of a credible and certified naturopath like Dr. Schmidt means that you can embrace your own health accountability and reap these rewards simply by adopting minor changes in your lifestyle. Getting back to nature is amazingly healing, a fact that has been known but not understood in the way that naturopaths have allowed us to.

Dr. Jana's story is a unique one. Whilst her parents may have been oil and water to one another, to her, they contributed and combined in the most amazing way to give her all of the tools that she needed to embrace the healing mentality and properties provided by nature. She will tell you more about it herself, but her life story is a fascinating one, and with us at TWC, she has found the perfect outlet for her remarkable talents.

Foster Coulson

Chapter 6

Nature Holds the Key to Transforming Health

Lessons Learned from The Native American Indians Jumping the Trail

> *"People at the time knew it was wrong.*
> *People at the time knew it was illegal.*
> *People at the time knew it was unconstitutional.*
> *And it happened anyway."*
> Dr. Amy H Sturgis on the 19th century American Trail of Tears

For thousands of years, forty thousand beautiful square Appalachian miles were the site of the Cherokee Nation, protected by a treaty that stated, "All people who have intruded or may hereafter intrude on lands reserved by the Cherokees shall be removed by the United States." However, in 1829 Andrew Jackson signed the Indian Removal Act, which rounded up thousands of Cherokees, removing them from their homes, sometimes even shackling and chaining them; forcing them to march at gunpoint. While we don't know precisely how many Cherokees died on this trek of approximately 2,200 miles to Oklahoma, scholars believe that somewhere between a quarter to one-third of the Cherokee

Nation was lost during this march to Oklahoma from the Eastern and Southern States that the Cherokees once inhabited.

In my story, I will share several generational blessings I have inherited from wise women and men in my family who have directed me in the heart of natural health. My great-grandmother, whom I only knew as Nitisi, was a Cherokee Native American healing woman. We understand that Grandmother Nitisi and her tribe jumped the Trail of Tears when people were dying from poor conditions and sickness. In addition, rumors of smallpox-laced blankets were being distributed to tribe members by the officials forcing them off their land. My great-grandmother had previously developed a concoction that she distributed during the winter months to tribe members. As I was told, none of them died on the trail from sickness; and they were able to secretly get off the trail and settle into the mountains of West Virginia. In 2019, I heard rumors of smallpox being a threat once again. An internal red flag went up when an infamous person in the mainstream media was filmed stating through an ominous smirk, that it would be terrible if smallpox got out, as it could decimate about forty percent of the population.

This was the same person who announced that there needed to be billions invested in research and development to protect us from the "next pandemic." And this was all before COVID-19 hit.

I was catapulted to research action over the potential smallpox concern. As I've done so many hundreds of nights during my career as a Naturopath, I found myself pouring over piles of books and researching late into the night, determined to learn of natural healing remedies for my tribe of people, which was then my family, friends and private naturopathic practice in Florida. My community has grown to encompass many more since then.

Recalling the Native American stories passed down from grandparents of the struggles and bravery in the face of adversity thrust upon them on the Trail of Tears, I am in awe of their resilience, strength, and determination to thrive. I am inspired with courage to speak up in truth, act with integrity, make my family proud, and continue the tradition of natural remedies for daily life as I guide my family in natural healing and strive for health freedom.

During some of my pajama-clad late-night research—armed with a favorite herbal tea and an insatiable desire for more information, I found documentation of other Native American tribes using the same or similar healing formulas as my Grandma Nitisi once used. In fact, with a relatively diligent search, you can find this information as well.

I discovered many accounts in history where Native American communities successfully used the same herbs and plants to protect from smallpox and other infirmities that Grandmother Nitisi used for her tribe. To my surprise, I also came across an NIH article that detailed the precise healing blend my grandmother had given to her Cherokee brethren so many decades ago.

There is a huge number of studies that support the effectiveness of therapies that originate from Native American practice. For example, below is the title and abstract that begins a well-known NIH study:

In Vitro Characterization of a Nineteenth Century Therapy for Smallpox

ABSTRACT: "In the nineteenth century, smallpox ravaged through the United States and Canada. At this time, a botanical preparation, derived from the carnivorous plant *Sarracenia purpurea*, was proclaimed as being a successful therapy for smallpox infections. The work described characterizes the anti-poxvirus activity associated with this botanical extract against vaccinia virus, monkeypox virus and variola virus, the causative agent of smallpox. Our work demonstrates the *in vitro* characterization of *Sarracenia purpurea* as the first effective inhibitor of poxvirus replication at the level of early viral transcription. With the renewed threat of poxvirus-related infections, our results indicate *Sarracenia purpurea* may act as another defensive measure against *Orthopoxvirus* infections."

Another article from Pub Med1865 is titled, "Report of the Trial of Sarracenia Purpurea, or the Pitcher Plant, in Small-Pox"

From Chemistry World: May 2012, "Rediscovered Native American Remedy Kills Poxvirus," and reads, "an old herbal remedy for treating smallpox that is thought to have been used by native Americans in the late 1800s has been rediscovered and found to kill the poxvirus."

From Research Gate: August 2020, "Herbal medicine used to treat smallpox in the 19th century found to halt viral replication in vitro."

From Frontiers 2020: "Pandemics and Traditional Plant-Based Remedies. A Historical-Botanical Review in the Era"

The list goes on and on of similar articles detailing the curative nature of Native American effective healing remedies for various illnesses. Upon securing the ingredients for the unique combination my family had used to protect from smallpox, a botanical blend was recreated. I also collaborated on a proprietary formulation for this health concern for my brave, amazing and dear friend, Dr. Stella Immanuel. Several other doctors reached out to me for advice on blending remedies for their "tribes" as well. While there is research and a claim by the NIH that this combination of plants works to protect and heal 100 percent of the viruses in that family, I choose not to make such a claim on any of my products for a variety of reasons both legally and philosophically. My hope is to empower, educate and assist people to live their most healthy life by using the very best resources nature has to offer and to confidently become their own health advocates.

Becoming A Profound Herald for Health Freedom

My name is Dr. Jana Schmidt and I'm a fourth-generation Natural Health Provider, like my Cherokee Great-grandmothers before me and my own mother, who lived a natural life as a "hippie" in a commune in Virginia for many years. I have sought divine guidance to share healing to thousands and even millions of people worldwide through my research, education, writing, healing herbs, supplements, combinations, teas and most of all dedication and passion. One of my goals is to carry on the blessings that have been generously given to me by God through generations of healing women and men before me with efficacy, hope, and love.

As some of you have heard me say from the stage at the Reawaken Tours in recent months, "For God has not given us a spirit of fear, but of power and of love and of a sound mind." I pray that we can embrace this truth, especially amid today's chaos.

My intention in this book and through my chapter is that you too will become a profound herald and achieve your own health sovereignty. I pray that you learn the natural healthy ways of our ancestors, develop effective ways to avoid illness, and have the ability to recover from devastating diseases. I pray your family will be healthier and stronger; not just in the body, but in mind and spirit as well. I pray that you will live a longer, more abundant life free from fear and the narrow confines of the big corporations whose sole interest in you is the profit you represent.

I encourage you to grasp the blessing of learning ways to partner with doctors that have your best interests at heart and become empowered to address common ailments and daily threats to prevent more serious illnesses from developing. Be open to learning about how God-given natural remedies contribute to living an abundantly healthy life. We are God-made. Therefore, God created remedies that correspond beautifully with our bodies. This is not a venture you need to take alone, I and many others are willing to help you on this empowering health journey.

The Flower Child

The year was 1972 and I stumbled into the little house in the woods on the Virginia hippie commune, where my mother raised me alongside friends and neighbors who were extended branches of my family.

I ran through the front door, my 5-year-old feet pattering on the wooden floors towards the kitchen where my mother and aunties were preparing food for dinner that night. My mother stood near the sink under a window where she had watched me gather eggs from the hen house. She saw my eyes fill with tears as I showed her the cut on my hand, received from a broken branch near the hen house and now bleeding over my hand onto the floor. She quickly whisked me up to the sink and held my hand under the cold running water, while my auntie cleaned the floor and grabbed a clean cloth for my hand.

My mother wrapped my hand and instructed me to find an aloe that had mature leaves and break off a whole leaf. My auntie took me by the other hand, and we went to the garden area in search of the perfect aloe leaf for my cut and some Chamomile for a calming tea. I broke off a small but full leaf and returned inside, where my mother opened the aloe and spread the soothing gel across the cut on my hand. I marveled at the soothing properties of the aloe plant. This wasn't the first, nor would it be the last time that a child would run into the house for help and be met by either my mom or a loving auntie who would simply guide us to the garden outside, calmly saying: "Grab peppermint leaves for your upset tummy" or "Pick some meadowsweet and lavender for your headache."

From the time I was five years old, my family - my community - taught and encouraged me to be a critical-thinking individual and my own health advocate. They taught me how to understand health cues my body would give and heal what ailed me with the right food, lifestyle, and herbs. I was not given Tylenol or ibuprofen, and fast-food was never on the menu for my meals. I didn't even taste an actual soda until I was about 14 years old—which, by the way, I did not enjoy. This was not surprising at all because I consumed little to no refined sugar.

However, my plates and pockets were regularly filled with fresh veggies, berries and herbs that I consumed like many of my peers ate candy. The garden was full of beautiful nutritious plants that made wholesome meals and delicious snacks.

I pause for a moment to reflect on two other generational blessings I haven't yet shared. There was Grandma Nitisi, my Native American healing woman and great-grandmother. There was my mother, who raised me in that hippie community in the 1970s, but I also carry a blessing from my maternal grandmother of a different and yet also impactful kind. Add to this my father, who as a physician modeled true care for his patients and especially me.

Around the same time as I was learning valuable ways of achieving natural health, at the age of 5, my maternal grandmother took me to church, where a Sunday School teacher told me that Jesus was always with me, always listening to me, and always engaging with what I had to say. As an only child, I was thrilled to have the Lord at my fingertips, waiting to hear my musings, my thoughts, my prayers, and my concerns at a moment's notice. At the age of 5, I began talking to Jesus every day and building an amazing relationship with Him.

The community was more than supportive of my interests and endeavors, including my newfound friend, Jesus. They thought it was creative that I had an "imaginary" friend. My family was kind, loving, caring, and generous and they loved watching me grow happily, feeling secure and fulfilled. Never once did somebody tell me to stop talking to Jesus. In fact, when I would respond that I was not talking to myself, but rather talking to Jesus, they would in turn respond, "Right On" or "Far Out Little One." I was always encouraged to sincerely express myself and grow intellectually, creatively, and spiritually. All these decades later I marvel at how many of those beautiful community members from the past have developed their own relationships with Jesus.

My father was also a big supporter of my health independence but from the allopathic side. In most ways, my parents were yin and yang. Dad was a Navy Seal corpsman who transitioned from the Navy after

Vietnam to become a physician. My mother was at home protesting the war when my father was serving in the Navy so, needless to say, their relationship was not the match they had hoped. Predictably, their lives soon went in different directions. However, I was still able to glean what was good in each of them and their lifestyles.

My father, as a physician, was like no doctor I had seen then or now. He was a wholesome triathlete who'd make rounds after hiking or biking for miles; giving patients care like they were his own family. I learned so much from his shining example of tireless, true dedication and exemplary health care.

Growing up, my father would often put me in a lab coat and have me complete rounds with him in his rural clinic. Tagging along, I would listen to him sincerely connect with each person and truly help them get well. Healing was everywhere when spending time with my dedicated father. He never turned down an opportunity to help people, and he would never turn away someone in need. I can remember many family dinners interrupted by a knock on the door by someone with an injury in need of help. My father also willingly made house calls any day or night of the week. He was an excellent example of caring for others. By bringing me into his work and world, I have always felt linked to my father's legacy of caring for people. In comparison to many of my peers, as I grew up, rather than consuming television programs and junk food during the afternoons, I consumed medical wisdom and empathy.

In addition, I had a family member who was a brilliant botanist and created a highly successful natural supplement company. From a young age, I observed him combine, analyze and certify ingredients for supplements, assessing what compounds went together and how they would work. From his work and willingness to share with me, I grew in my understanding of plants from a scientific viewpoint. Since then, I have continued this love of botany and discovering the miraculous healing powers of plants.

In the community with my mother, the protective and grounding time spent with my grandparents, and the wholesome and engaging life with my father, I was treated as a valued member of the family: as a true individual. I was not treated as merely a child; I was honored as a bright, contributing person to conversations and decisions, and regarded as a valued member of the community. In nearly every way, I had a childhood that built my confidence, filled me with joy, and prepared me for the future.

Something that resonated with me (then and now) was the emphasis on outdoor time and laughter. Patch Adams, whom I still treasure today, was our community doctor and he emphasized these important activities in the process of healing. I knew I was a witness to the truly miraculous ways in which he helped and healed people, but it was not until much later that I realized the magnitude of a blessing he had been in my life and in so many others. I recall fondly that he used to say that laughter is an integral part of healing. I grew to understand the scientific accuracy of this statement; laughter helps raise dopamine levels, assists with digestion, and wards off depression—not to mention the benefit laughing with friends has on building a sense of community and intimacy among people. We are finding, with an ever-growing amount of evidence, that isolation is one of the most egregious issues of the pandemic.

Patch even assisted my grandmother break free from medications that were prescribed to her which possessed too many negative side effects. He helped her to holistically restore her health and I am forever grateful. Between my father, mother, aunties, grandparents, and Patch, it was no surprise that when I expressed the desire to become a doctor they encouraged me toward Naturopathic medicine. This was an important decision, one that that was in the making for many years. As a result, I have penned my own book, *Growing Up Flower Child,* which details my childhood in the midst of the Vietnam War, communal living, and health wisdom journey from my childhood perspective.

"They're" Not in It For The Healing...

Like any flower child, I am faithful to focus on love and light in both my public and private conversations. Almost daily, I have the opportunity to embrace a scared and hopeless person, reminding them that God is the provider of everything we need. I often spread encouragement to those that I speak to publicly and via email who are seeking guidance, telling them that:

"There's no evil man can create that our God cannot overcome."

Optimistic and gentle as I feel and present myself, there is a profound urgency to my message. A scientific study conducted many years ago, which I'll share in the next section, subconsciously fuels me and partially illustrates the reason I devote so much of my time engaging people to be empowered advocates of health freedom. I have felt deep down - from the time I was a little barefoot 5-year-old picking peppermint for my tummy ache - that what I need to live a remarkably healthy life can be found in what God provides; in particular, in the beautiful and curative plants. It turns out that my Great-grandmother Nitisi knew this well two hundred years ago.

Scientists working on behalf of pharmaceutical companies are also aware of elements in nature that can cheaply, non-invasively, and effectively address diseases.

Enter: The Birch Tree.

While walking in the forest, University of Minnesota Chemistry Professor Robert Carlson one day noticed that everything on the forest floor was deteriorating much faster than birch bark. Whilst making this observation, he was struck with an idea that could have changed our world. As a result, Carlson became a pioneer researcher of birch bark, particularly a form of the bark processed into pellets called betulin.

His first lab test showed that betulin may successfully treat herpes. Naturally, he was compelled to continue his studies.

In 2006, a factory in Two Harbors, Minnesota, began extracting a natural chemical from the bark of birch trees to meet global demand for more natural compounds and chemicals, as well as gain access to healing properties that have the potential to fight disease. The laboratory learned that 90 percent of the trees used in paper mills are wasted; burned in boilers instead of being used. Now, there was a better solution: birch bark formerly incinerated could be used in medicines and cosmetics.

Birch bark betulin wasn't synthetic, and because the process of extracting betulin could be patented, nature cannot be patented. Just like my Great-grandmother's concoction for curing smallpox on the Trail of Tears has now been widely researched and accepted, birch has been reverently held by Native Americans as an element of both medicinal and spiritual importance.

Finally, the pharmaceutical company that paid for the birch bark betulin studies killed them off because it could not be made stable enough to patent. Sadly, birch bark demonstrated promising evidence that could be used to help heal skin cancer and other dermatological ailments. Over twenty-five years ago, armed with this knowledge, and the healing herb lessons gleaned from those before me and my past mentor Dr. Philip Fritchie, ND/ Master Herbalist, I developed a salve years ago that, while I won't claim any guarantees, is shown to help the skin benefit from the healing powers of birch bark and fourteen other incredible botanicals.

Censorship

Steeped in the naturals, I've long been a fan of natural botanicals instead of pharmaceutical medications. For instance, I chose to take Quercetin in lieu of hydroxychloroquine. The natural alternative to ivermectin that I prefer is sweet wormwood. I have naturally helped over five thousand people, none of whom died from COVID-19 or even went into the hospital for COVID-19 treatments.

Every day, we make a choice for our immune systems, and among the best of those choices is the decision to seek natural preventatives and healing substances for our bodies in lieu of chemicals, whenever possible. For example, bee pollen is an example of God's perfect whole food multivitamin, white willow bark, and aspen bark contain salicylic acid akin to aspirin, whilst garlic is an incredible antibacterial, rose hips are one of the best sources of Vitamin C, and sunshine is our best source of Vitamin D.

You may be surprised to learn that pharmaceutical companies create many medications from natural plant ingredients. They often use natural elements for the foundations of the medications and then add chemical substances to the base plant and/ or take something away from the natural plant to make a pharmaceutical medicine. For instance, in Silymarin, a drug made to help protect and regenerate the liver, the active ingredient is derived from the milk thistle plant. Milk thistle itself cannot be patented, but an altered active ingredient of milk thistle can.

Amazingly, I recently read a study that proved that dirt can work in a manner like Prozac—in some cases, better than Prozac. Touching and breathing the tiny microbes in the soil act as an antidepressant and the benefits can be felt for up to three weeks. I am regularly in the garden tending to the plants with bare hands. No wonder I am so happy all the time.

Below are some examples of natural herbs and plants and their restorative properties:

**COMMON PHARMACEUTICAL
AND PLANT BASES**

ASPIRIN	WHITE WILLOW OR ASPEN BARK
TAMIFLU	STAR ANISE
VALIUM	VALERIAN
QUININE	CINCHONA
TAXOL	YEW PINE
SILYMARIN	MILK THISTLE
EPHEDRINE	EPHDRA
HESPERIDIN	CITRIS
DANTHRON	CASSIA
L-DOPA	MUCUNA

Generally, companies are patenting an element that is primarily a natural ingredient or formulation of ingredients, altering in some way the natural botanical by adding manmade elements, and thereby patenting what could have been a natural formulation without the potential numerous side effects often resulting from manmade versions of the remedy.

It's A Fight To Do What's Right For the Patient

My amazing husband and I have raised our children holistically, mainly in sunny Hawaii and Florida where we homeschooled them surrounded by large gardens, with chickens and bees. They, like me in my childhood, have embraced a life that emphasizes health wisdom and helping others. I often joke that my sons are all qualified to give my signature stage lectures on my behalf. As an international pilot, my husband has given us all the opportunities to travel and embrace the world. This has given us all the gift of a worldview of life, love, health, and healing.

Our oldest son is, like his Mom and Dad, an ordained minister. He's a "Musicianary"; a missionary (Creative World Missions) and a musician (Coastland) whose non-profit organization uses music and missions to bridge the gap to enter places that otherwise would be impossible. He has teamed up with others to help rescue children from the darkest, most desperate places all over the world.

Our middle son is a brilliant shining light in the much-needed world of advertising and is a musical genius, whilst our youngest is currently in the police academy, dedicating his life to helping others and securing our freedoms. All are living glowing examples of brilliance, kindness, and radiant health; inside and out.

A naturopathic doctor in the State of Florida isn't all sunshine and palm trees though. In fact, Florida is a big American Medical Association and pharmaceutical state. Not only is the State of Florida a constant challenge due to regulations, but the allopathic world in general doesn't always want to "play nicely" with naturopaths. There are few cheers when the people I help walk into their doctor's office and tell them that I've assisted them in a plan to improve their health with natural remedies and a change in diet.

Over the past few decades, I have lost count of the times medical doctors have rejected the opportunity to help their patients break free from over-medication. It's heartbreaking to know that these individuals would experience better care if all modalities of health and healing were offered to them and if a variety of doctors were willing to work together. This is part of the change I am honored to be a part of, where MDs who have undergone valuable training and knowledge are paired with wise NDs creating a powerful combination for the betterment of all their patients.

Although the State of Florida doesn't allow naturopathic doctors to practice independently, I'm an ordained minister which allows me to continue my work as my ministry—which it most certainly is. When I meet with an individual, I spend at least one hour in our first consultation. I see each person as a puzzle, where my goal is to gather as many pieces as I can in order to see the big picture.

By contrast, in a consultation limited to fifteen minutes (as is often the norm), crucial details to the puzzle can be missed. People often come to see me because they're exhausted and want to be heard; they need a life change from masking symptoms to arriving at healing from their ailments. The more time spent with detailed questions asked, the more likely we are to discover what is missing and begin the healing process. With The Wellness Company, we are committed to bringing medical professionals together from both the allopathic and naturopathic approaches. We are dedicated to harmoniously working together to help people get well and stay well.

I am not comfortable with the wartime language and name-calling rampant in some arenas of fighting for freedom. I must admit, though, it's calling it *fighting* for a reason. It only monetarily behooves the pharmaceutical companies if people remain sick. Fighting for your right to healthy choices and avenues of healing is of paramount importance.

Please do not misunderstand me; I know and am grateful for modern medical advancements. However, I am not impressed with the overuse of medications and over-testing. I much prefer to get to the root of the problem and help a person heal from sickness than to simply mask a symptom or rack up a bill with lab after lab test. Sometimes, medications and labs are very necessary for certain situations and sometimes they are not. It takes a true professional to know the difference. I am honored to know and work with such doctors; ones who care first and foremost for their patients' healing, their futures, and their overall wellbeing. We have an arsenal of God-given tools from nature and life-saving pharmaceuticals that we are using to ensure health wins for everyone.

The Intervention

In 2020, a psychologist with whom I shared an office, along with an MD, sat me down over one of many lunches we shared together.

"I'm worried about you. Worried that you're getting involved with the wrong people and they're going to take advantage of you," she said, taking my hands, concern in her voice.

I reminded her of the need for freedom and the importance of making choices with informed consent.

"We don't have the information we need to recommend, let alone take, this shot," I told her, showing as much care and respect as I could.

Soon after, I was disassociated from that office, even though I'd worked harmoniously for several years with an MD and that "concerned" psychologist.

Although the MD and I have not spoken since, that psychologist and I are still close and work in the realm of stress and trauma. After she experienced problems with her second shot, I reminded her that she had not been properly informed.

It hurts me that those colleagues were wrongly informed and continued to recommend an experimental gene therapy in lieu of natural remedies when I and so many others achieved such remarkable success helping people heal and stay well naturally.

Today, my new office-mates are a group of freedom-loving Godly patriots. I still help people in person and over the phone. I'm endlessly passionate and highly successful in helping couples with fertility. I am currently writing a book called *The Fertility Formula* that gathers the collective years of wisdom in the realm of fertility. Over the past twenty-six years, I have been blessed to help couples with a wide range of infertility issues, learn natural ways to conceive, and carry a healthy baby to full term.

I believe health is God's design for our lives, which is what compels me to persist in recommending natural ways to heal bodies and help couples achieve optimal health and optimal chances of conceiving. For instance, did you know that a cell phone in a man's pants pocket can reduce his sperm count by 75 percent? Did you also know that WiFi radiation is equally harmful to women—not an ideal environment for someone wanting to have children?

I am moved by God's assurance that "the one who is in you is greater than the one who is in the world."

The Shift

In 2021, when I saw many MD friends suffer because they were not able to practice medicine, they were being forced to corroborate a false narrative, violate their Hippocratic oaths, and even asked to inject dangerous experimental shots into their bodies against their will to keep their jobs. My heart broke to watch dedicated, brilliant doctors forced out of their hospitals, groups, and practices due to their diligence in bringing the best-informed healthcare possible. In the fall of 2020, I was asked to join a prominent doctors' group bringing medical freedom information to the world, partially because I was not censored from helping people. Natural sources are not controlled by pharmaceuticals, hospitals or insurance companies. So far, no one can patent sunshine.

Doctors have been called, above all else, to help and not harm people. Censoring some of the most well-respected doctors in the world because they question mass media narratives is obviously harmful.

If you're like me, you experienced a profound awakening when you read about something like the birch bark covered-up data or even when you first realized that COVID-19 illness was being used for control, power, and greed. It is important to question, research, read, and stay close to trusted sources. I believe the deception started a long time ago and the deception continues.

Broken Commitment

At events where I am invited to speak, I meet many people whose friendships continue to grow as our paths cross in the fight for medical freedom. Some of the connections, whom I fondly refer to as "Godly patriots," invited me to join a group of doctors and business-minded people to collaborate on building a better system to care for people; real health care, not "sick care."

Joining a professional team forging a new way of healthcare sounded too good to be true. In this group, the MDs, NDs, PAs, and nurses were led to believe that we would all work together to build a platform for all-encompassing care that integrated both allopathic and naturopathic.

I chose to trust this group of people, although there were people I did not know very well among those I already trusted. Sadly, after months of tirelessly devoting my time, knowledge, and resources, this organization crumbled . Now, I may not be that business savvy, but I could clearly see that when numbers become the focus over the people, problems arise. To my dismay, I learned that not all who profess medical freedom are able to do what it takes to accomplish that end. Even as the "freedom medical organization" was crumbling, I was still speaking at events.

At one such event, I was happily reunited with some true, dear friends in the medical freedom movement: Dr. Heather Gessling and Dr. Jen VanDeWater. They were bubbling with excitement about a new project underway and underwraps. I was intrigued but respectful of the confidentiality. Just twelve hours prior that company had dissolved all its contracts and fundamentally ceased to exist. When Dr. Heather Gessling asked me if I was committed by contract to any other company, I happily shared what had happened twelve hours prior. That night, Dr. Heather called me to share the vision of The Wellness Company.

The Blessing

People often ask me what my hope for the future is.

I pray that all will have the resources to grow food that nourishes our minds, bodies, and souls with dense nutrients that are provided by the plants.

As a Naturopath, it is important to me that the whole body is balanced through nutrition, supplementation, and lifestyle while delivered with excellence and integrity. For too long, these have been separated or not addressed at all in health and healing. I've at last found a team that aligns with these goals.

When The Wellness Company approached me, I was captivated by Foster's incredible drive to create and his brilliant mind for business, even well before The Wellness Company. I met Dr Gessling, Dr Amerling and Dr Vandewater in the summer of 2021. Friendships grew alongside my high esteem and appreciation for their dedicated work for true patient care and health freedom. When they invited me to join them and contribute to The Wellness Company, I felt honored to be a part of an incredible team that embraces essential facets of patient care that have long been so important to me.

As member of the Integrative Therapeutic Board with The Wellness Company, I look forward to continuing to use my passion and knowledge for teaching, continuing to develop proprietary blends, and writing more articles that inform and empower people to become grounded in natural healing so that they feel comfortable partnering with their doctor to become well and stay healthy.

The future of health freedom looks bright and it includes a deep desire that cares about your health, providing useful information that you can easily incorporate into your lifestyle for a solid health foundation. This is a foundation that you can share with others and teach your family to continue the movement for health freedom. This is what you will discover from our team of remarkable doctors at TWC.

I continue to write blogs and articles, make videos and podcasts to continually share health freedom updates because the world is ever-changing and I want to help my tribe stay informed.

Remember that humanity has battled through a variety of illnesses and afflictions throughout history. A cursory internet search will readily illustrate how many diseases were handled through accurate scientific information, adapting lifestyles, and the incorporation of natural remedies.

We don't have to be afraid of what is around the corner or succumb to the growing hurricanes of fear that are falsely swept through our daily lives. Rather, we can find strength by simply remaining grounded by God, informed, and prepared. We at The Wellness Company are honored to be a driving force of health information, health care, and health freedom.

Blessings for Abundant Health and True Freedom,

Dr. Jana Schmidt

Chapter Six Takeaways

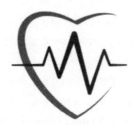

An essential part of embarking on your own positive health journey, free from the constraints and corruption of the Biopharmaceutical Complex, then the best way is to embrace the healing power that is found in the very ground we walk.

Who would have known about the restorative properties of dirt? Have you ever heard of the healing power of birch bark? I know I hadn't before now. The world is a big place, and it is our belief that we have only scratched the surface of what nature has to offer. We intend, through the wisdom and help of Dr. Schmidt, to advance this field of knowledge and to create supplements that can be brought to the market—not squashed and killed as they are now because they are "not profitable enough."

Nature is, I believe, one of the keys to removing the shackles of insurance-led care and ceasing feeding the bottom line of cash-cow hospitals.

Many doctors will agree that prevention is better than healing, and the best way to prevent the onset of many chronic illnesses. The earlier you embark on your health-positive journey the better, and we are to help start the process.

The list provided in this chapter of plants that can be found in the wild and their healing properties is not exhaustive. Naturopaths like Dr. Schmidt can help you discover many more, and it is so easy to take the kids and head out and forage for these. If your life is a bit busy though and the time to do so is hard to come by, then there are many supplements available that can help bring those benefits to you.

As with all of these things though, do your due diligence. Only buy supplements you can trust, and that are what they say they are. The Marketplace we are looking to create will help to do this for you, but don't just wait for us, join a tribe and seize the initiative now.

Foster Coulson

Conclusion

A Call for Connection

"Society is collapsing, and people are starting to recognize that the reason they feel like they're mentally ill is that they're living in a system that's not designed to suit the human spirit."

Russell Brand

I began this book with a story of how 2020 brought me to a crisis moment in my psyche because I know I'm not alone; you and I together faced our demons, whether internal or externally. One thing is for sure: we'll never be the same. For a period of time, human connection eroded. More than a virus, more than the myriad of theories as to why things were the way they were, nothing sickened me more to watch than that loss of human connection. Seeing news stories of or images of children visiting parents and grandparents only through Zoom, if at all… of all the upheaval in all of our lives over the past two years, these are the moments that are most illustrative of my own purpose: to be a uniting force for humanity.

Following the events of 2020 and 2021, the medical community at once became busier than ever, but it wasn't always in the best interest of patients. That's why you've read this book. You've seen that medicine has come to a turning point; we can either emerge wiser, stronger, and more determined, or we can allow the system to continue in the tyrannical, corporation-focused way it has been run.

Think of All We've Gained from the "Pandemic"

The healthcare professionals and medical freedom fighters here at The Wellness Company chose to take action. We've dedicated ourselves to overcoming a system that doesn't serve patients. By picking up this book, you can count yourself among those freedom fighters.

We've taken the time in this book to illustrate clearly how perverse the forces guiding our doctors and pharmacists hands have been. The darkness predates COVID-19 by decades, and it won't be immediately rectified. Once associations could be purchased by corporations, such as Dr. Richard Amerling illustrated in Chapter Five with the example of the American Heart Association, our medical system began to crumble. This system became focused on sick-care versus well-care; even over-prescribing to line the deep pockets of insurance and pharmaceutical corporations to the detriment of patients. However, the focus in this book never was to beat a dead horse or perpetuate the analysis of a broken system. Hopefully, what you've really taken away from this book is hope.

Unlike Dr. Amerling or Dr. Risch, who had for decades kept their fingers on the pulse of the degradation and destruction of American Medicine, many of us have become newly aware of the corruption of our medical system. During this time, we have remembered what matters, most especially with regard to community and intimacy. The people or powers that are wreaking havoc behind closed doors have succeeded not just in the premature deaths of hundreds of thousands of people, but they have taken away the very thing that makes life worth living.

The events of the past three years have sparked a profound awakening.

Happily, society is now waking up.

The six doctors in this book, who have had otherwise illustrious careers, were secretly being manipulated behind the scenes. Upon that awakening, we don't emerge with hard hearts, we emerge aligned for justice and a mission bigger than serving local patients. We have presented you with a blueprint for rewriting the entire system from the ground up.

Even as I write this, our Pharmacy Department has just enrolled a Nevada-based compounding pharmacy in our Wellness Pharmacy program. Now, people in the Las Vegas area as well as across forty-eight U.S. States where Partell is licensed will have a financially stable compounding pharmacy they can trust. Partell is partnered with and supported by The Wellness Company team to continue in their comprehensive patient continuum of care design and resistance to corporate greed and manipulation in the pharmaceutical industry. It is my ambition that within three years we will have two thousand Wellness Company supported pharmacies just like Partell Pharmacy to meet your needs.

Sometimes, awakening is a gentle stretch. Other times it's more like a bucket of ice in the face. I am not a doctor, but purpose seems to know how to get our attention when it needs us, and it's got mine. I suspect that if you've made it this far and you're still reading, it's got yours, too.

Welcome to the awakening. There is no snooze button.

Wellness Includes Happiness

Happiness is a critical part of your health, and alongside our Marketplace, The Well, Pharmacy, and Virtual Medicine services, we are committed to your overall psychological wellness, too.

How do you feel?

When your doctor is running down a list of questions from a script they received from their corporate medical overlords, are they taking the time to ask whether or not you're happy? Should they?

Maybe you have been completing yoga and meditation for years but you still find yourself struggling with pain or depression. What does your supplement regimen look like? It's about trial and error. Commit to finding, as I have, the formula that brings you wellness. I have found mine in eating home cooked meals using organic ingredients, a regular exercise routine, infrared sauna, meditation and a daily supplement routine. But what works for me may not work for you. That's where we're here to help.

My colleague Dr. Schmidt points out that simply putting your bare feet in living soil is more powerful than Prozac, and she understands the science to prove it. When you begin supplementing (or grounding down barefoot into your garden), be sure to take the five minutes it requires to find pharmaceutical-grade supplements versus the made-in-China sawdust that hasn't been third-party tested and does not do what it claims to do.

Find companies like The Wellness Company, or others, with products that have been third-party tested so that you can put the most optimal thing into your body. If your body is a temple - as so many world religions and philosophies believe - don't desecrate it. You wouldn't put sand in the gas tank or sub-par oil in an Italian sports car, so pay special attention to the sources of your supplements, nutraceuticals, or pharmaceuticals.

Perhaps this week you focus on spirituality and next week you focus on lifting heavier weights or performing more reps in your workout. Personally, I enjoy taking phone calls while trekking up a steep hill near my house for cardio training. Perhaps the ideal motivation for you is the freedom to live a healthy life while eliminating all tracking, point-keeping, scales, and comparisons.

In society, we receive a flood of dopamine from screens, social media, and the physical gratification of clicking buttons and notifications. From this flood of dopamine comes addiction. When you get just enough of what you want, you can train your brain to stay motivated without getting overstimulated; you get steady drips without the flood.

An Awakening of The Heart Through Purpose

> *"The worst part of being strong is that nobody asks if you're okay.*
> *It's okay to ask for help."*
> *Sergeant Major (Ret.) Mark Spicer, author of "Outdance The Devil"*

The healing and awakening journey we are all on starts in the heart. I've resolved a good majority of my own health challenges, and it wasn't because I work alongside pathologists, epidemiologists, cardiologists, and nephrologists, or because I know people trained in immunology and biology. All the science aside, I'm human. If I can overcome the bad habits that beget bad health, you can, too. Digging into technical papers engages our heads, but real change comes when our hearts come online. Looking at my wife and children reminds me that I want to be in the game for the long haul. Technical papers don't motivate me to be well, but connecting with the things and people I love do. There's a saying that the cure for addiction is not sobriety, but community. Resilience is not achieved alone. I couldn't agree more, and that's why The Well, a place for connection with other awakened health warriors like yourself, is probably my favorite TWC initiative.

However, we must first disconnect to reconnect. Our lives and brains follow habits that have formed into neural networks in our brains. We reach for ice cream when we're stressed or we scroll social media to connect... which actually leaves us feeling more isolated and less secure in ourselves and our success. Disconnecting from old habits and isolating activities is no small feat; to be successful, we must commit to a process of rewiring our brains. This involves rejecting the pastimes that have been designed to make us consumers of content in favor of intimacy and connection within our communities, families and our bodies. From that place of reconnection, we align with ourselves and our tribes; the people in our lives who are eager to support us.

This place of connection has many names: in yoga, it is the sacral chakra; in health, it's the social immune system. Whatever you call it, and however it comes to life for you, you achieve connection by tuning into our communities, paying attention to our partners, and surrendering to the flow of creative hobbies that stimulate our minds and create new neural pathways.

The doctors in this book explain a lot from the stage in terms that are technical, but your responsibility is to take that knowledge and run with it, growing and developing your own wisdom. Wisdom comes when we ignite the heady stuff with creative energy and align our hearts with it. The heart awakening, and bringing with it your sense of purpose, is where real change occurs.

You Have Permission to Be Well

My own intention with this story can be summarized in a single word: permission.

You have permission to heal. You have permission to be fully alive, creatively ignited, and deeply connected to the world around you. You have permission to be disappointed in the world and the people in it, but you also have permission to be free from fear.

Lauryn Maloney Gepfert is a kinesiologist and neurofunctional healer who runs an organization called The Neurofunctional Institute (NFI). Through NFI, Gepfert helps men and women who have been paralyzed restore movement with the power of their thoughts.

A few years ago, I might have not understood, but I now recognize that she has a pioneering philosophy about changing one's life and body by changing one's mind. She reports that one of the most unyielding barriers to healing is the fact that people do not permit their bodies to do what they are designed to do. Our bodies are designed to heal, and that healing starts with a thought. Creating the optimal conditions to allow healing to occur starts with giving your body permission to heal.

Now, go grab a whiteboard marker and walk over to your bathroom mirror. Write these words:

You have permission to heal

Speak those words with authority over your body and mind every day. Don't use the word "I" have permission to heal, that only serves to dissociate the thought from the body. Speak to your own body, using the word "you." You have permission to heal. You have the power to heal within you. You deserve to heal, and we need you in fighting form for the road ahead.

On Fear

I've taken a lot of heat for my association with Zev Zelenko, who infamously used the term "poison death shot" when referring to the investigative gene-based therapy also called the COVID-19 vaccine. Other doctors have called the COVID-19 shot program "tyranny with a needle" or the "needle in every arm program," the "clotshot," or even more descript and disturbing terms and images.

All clever monikers aside, people are scared of what the next wave or variant will be. Although some doctors believe that future variants of COVID-19 prove to be demonstrably less virulent over time, other highly respected virologists, such as Dr. Geert Vanden Bosshe, Ph.D., DVM, warn that "the virus will win."

Even if people are not scared of the next wave or variant that's unleashed either by man or lab, they *are* scared of the unknown. They are scared of fear-mongering and the nervousness none of us could escape for two years. That stress categorically weakens our immune systems.

People do feel tyrannized; we're all waking up to flagrant abuses of power around us. People do feel violated and victimized; I have heard innumerable stories of men and women losing their jobs and even their children due to mandates that don't work for every patient in every situation, culture, religious persuasion, or stage of life. And finally, people do fear "the clotshot," or any number of the myriad of complications from potentially taking or from having already taken the investigative gene-based therapy called a COVID-19 vaccine.

But what are we really scared of?

We're scared of losing our freedom. We are scared of losing the right to make decisions for our bodies… or not to. We're scared of losing our right to choose. We are scared of losing the freedom to opt-out of an experimental treatment, the freedom to work, to socialize. The freedom to breathe fresh air.

Medical institutions promoting one-size-fits-all answers to anything is scary, as Drs Amerling and Risch have illustrated.

It wasn't until I sat with all this scary stuff and took the time to process it that I conquered and transmuted it. Sit with the words I've just written and the fear it strikes in you. See the faces of loved ones sitting in hospital hells alone; even dying there with nobody around. Feel the anger and heat building behind your eyes as you read those words.

YES. That's why we're here. That's why we throw around these hard-hitting terms about tyranny and clots and violation. We're not melodramatic. We're certainly not conspiracy theorists. We're ready to fight, and there is something righteous about that. Don't let anybody tell you otherwise.

You have permission to fight. As you process everything you and I are about, find healthy habits and hobbies that act as therapy, like Dr. VanDeWater and her garden paradise; transmute that anger into righteous action.

The Next Wave Is Brave.

Finding Your Voice

Now that you have permission to be angry, how do you make an impact without perpetuating more fear? The Wellness Company is filled with individuals who have made sacrifices and experienced losses as a result of their stance on healthcare, particularly off the back of the pandemic. Dr. McCullough lost three professorships.

We're not deterred; we're activated. We're activated because there's a greater good that we are trying to achieve, and we will continue to speak out. For every detractor, there are ten thousand supporters, as my colleague Dr. McCullough pointed out. When, like us, you find a voice that comes from a place of compassion and care, you'll catch more flies, so to speak.

When interviewing Risch and McCullough, they each pointed out something that amazed me; they are rarely, if ever, criticized by anybody reputable. Their points, although labeled by largely unqualified or ignorant sources as conspiracy theories, are backed by science. Perhaps these doctors have lost clients or contracts for their controversial views, but these views aren't theories; they're based in objective, empirical realities. That's why you and I keep listening.

The Wellness Company doctors now travel around the country and the world where pathologists, oncologists, physicians, and radiation technicians are seeing complications and cancers at a rate we have never seen before. One of our colleagues attended a conference call very recently with a large group in New York, where one doctor reported seeing record numbers of 20-30 year-olds coming in with breast cancer, often just weeks after their boosters. The Chair of Oncology at a large hospital in Florida reached out to that same colleague and said, "Hey doc, thanks for speaking out. I usually see an aggressive brain cancer and a young patient about every decade or so. I've seen five in the last month after the boosters." A doctor from Ireland who's been in medicine for thirty years shared with us that he is seeing patients who have been cancer free for up to five years suddenly take a booster and wind up with a stage four disease again. We don't want this to be happening, but this is what brilliant scientists are observing. So we won't stop talking about it.

It's because of our purpose that people keep listening. When you find your own voice, it's from that purpose-driven place that you will have the most impact.

Along the way, take a lesson from motivational speaker Jim Rohn and surround yourself with people who model the presence you want to have in this world. Don't forget to humbly receive praise when you do impact others. Time and again somebody tells the doctors in this team that they have saved their father or sibling; which fuels them to hop on the next plane or spend another weekend at a conference helping people understand what we're up against—not to perpetuate fear, but so they, too, can become teachers.

Take the models and lessons we share with TWC and become a teacher in your community. You have the power to save just as many lives as we do. Truly, we can't do this work alone; we need your voice, too.

The Next Wave Is Brave

Our doctors collectively receive thousands of messages every day. They aspire to respond to every one of them, which is why we've created TWC Media, a place where we can make 1+1=11. A trusted place for answers. By aligning with some of the most distinguished scientists and compassionate physicians on the planet, our output increases exponentially.

It's been said that you can lead a horse to water, but you cannot make it drink. But, when people taste the water, it becomes their journey. The family of medical freedom fighters includes you; you're an individual and an important disciple of wellness.

With so many purposeful freedom fighters they find the ability to transmute their anger, disgust, or fear into love. Fueled with purpose, they don't have time to scroll social media and self-consciously compare themselves to others or read yet another article that articulates the same terrifying point as the last four they read or saw tweeted. Moving from fear involves getting so busy with purpose that you don't have time to worry.

Your courage begets courage in others. Your purposeful life inspires others to live more meaningfully. Your meaningful action provides the blueprints for others to take action.

Now, come march with us.

Foster Coulson

Join The Wellness Revolution

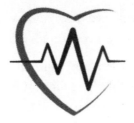

What would it mean to live in a world with medical freedom? What would that look like for our parents, your children, and for yourself? Help us construct a new system in place of the old systems that are now crumbling.

Here's how you share the Wellness Revolution with your community.

1) **Read about our bravery muse** Dr. Zev Zelenko by visiting www.ZevsBook.com where you'll experience the thrilling, page-turning account of how one man started a movement that united medical freedom fighters to save millions of lives.

2) **Give this book to your doctor.** Email support@twc.health if you'd like to purchase bulk copies for family, friends, and local healthcare professionals.

3) **Give this book to your library.** Your library isn't going to seek out this "controversial" blueprint to a wellness revolution and

medical freedom, so supply it for them. Perhaps your town has free libraries in strategic locations; supply those free libraries with *The Next Wave Is Brave* so that we can get the message out to our community.

4) **Ask** Barnes and Noble or other Bookstores to order *The Next Wave Is Brave*. Once enough people demand *The Next Wave Is Brave*, bookstores will begin carrying the book and giving it increasingly more desirable shelf space.

5) **Write an amazing five-star review** wherever you purchased this book and/or wherever you love buying books.

6) **Elevate** your supplement regimen with Wellness Company Vitality and Signature products. Our supplement lines each give back to a charity so that you'll feel good fueling your body with high-quality ingredients while also supporting a cause that elevates the world.

7) **Join the Campfire**: visit us at twc.health where you'll connect with other like-minded wellness warriors.

8) Follow TWC on all social platforms.

Facebook:
https://www.facebook.com/TheWellnessCompany.health

Twitter:
https://twitter.com/twc_health

Gab:
https://gab.com/thewellnesscompany

Truth Social:
https://truthsocial.com/login

Gettr:
https://gettr.com/user/thewellnesscompany

Instagram:
https://www.instagram.com/twc.health/

Telegram:
https://t.me/thewellnesscompany

YouTube:
https://www.youtube.com/channel/
UCDdyHqmkbqRKzQqK5xje1kg

LinkedIn:
https://www.linkedin.com/company/twc-wellness-company/

9) Share your #NextWaveIsBrave moments on social media. This is how other UnCaged badasses will find you. We're strong on our own... but we're even stronger together!

Yours in Medical Freedom,

The Wellness Company Family

Author's Note

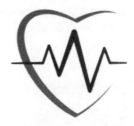

This book isn't over yet—our journey to medical freedom is just beginning. Please join us at www.twc.health where we will continue to provide more information and updates about the fight against tyranny by the hospital corporations, pharma, and other bad actors in healthcare. We eagerly await your presence in our Wellness Pharmacies, Wellness Telemedicine, Wellness Media, and Wellness Marketplace. Thank you for hearing our stories and supporting the movement to liberate and heal the world.

The Wellness Company
www.twc.health

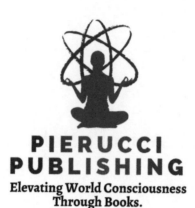

PIERUCCI
PUBLISHING
**Elevating World Consciousness
Through Books.**

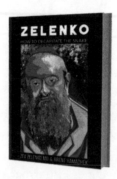

Zelenko: How to Decapitate the Serpent

"In a small way, this book is a metaphor for each of us to continue to hold up the arms of a great man – Dr. Zev Zelenko – and, like Aaron and Hur, keep his arms lifted in the battle against the terrorists in lab coats until We the People can win the battle and the day for a brighter future for humanity."
Dr. David E. Martin

Available now at www.ZelenkoBook.com